Alzheimer's Disease

ALZHEIMER'S DISEASE

A Practical Guide for Families and Other Caregivers

Judah L. Ronch

Foreword by William Van Ornum

Crossroad | *New York*

1993

The Crossroad Publishing Company
370 Lexington Avenue
New York, NY 10017

Copyright © 1989 by Judah L. Ronch
Foreword Copyright © 1989 by William Van Ornum

All rights reserved. No part of this book may be reproduced,
stored in a retrieval system, or transmitted, in any form
or by any means, electronic, mechanical, photocopying, recording,
or otherwise, without the written permission of
The Crossroad Publishing Company.

Printed in the United States of America

Library of Congress Cataloging-in-Publication Data

Ronch, Judah, L.
  Alzheimer's disease : a practical guide for families and other
caregivers / Judah L. Ronch ; foreword by William Van Ornum.
    p. cm.
  ISBN 0–8264–0500–2; ISBN 0–8245–1284–7 (pbk.)
1. Alzheimer's disease—Patients—Care. 2. Alzheimer's disease—
Patients—Family relationships. I. Title. II. Series.
RC523.R65 1989
618.97'683—dc19   88–26818
                                                                                                     CIP

To Robin

Contents

Foreword by William Van Ornum, Ph.D.   9

Preface   11

Acknowledgments   13

CHAPTER 1 | The Impact of Alzheimer's Disease on the Victim   19

CHAPTER 2 | Separation and Loss in Alzheimer's Disease: The Impact on the Family   33

CHAPTER 3 | Communicating with the Demented Elderly Person   70

CHAPTER 4 | Counseling Older Persons   76

CHAPTER 5 | Counselors Have Feelings, Too   93

CHAPTER 6 | Understanding, Explaining, and Intervening When Problem Behavior Occurs   109

CHAPTER 7 | Assessing Service Needs, Finding Resources, and Making Referrals   143

CHAPTER 8 | Counseling and Residential Long-term Care Placement of the Alzheimer's Victim   155

Appendix A   Alzheimer's and Other Dementias   170

Appendix B   Care Services for Dementia Patients   190

Notes   193

Bibliography   202

Alzheimer's Disease

Judah L. Ronch, author of *Alzheimer's Disease,* is a gerontological psychologist—one specializing in the emotional and developmental concerns of older persons.

Dealing with Alzheimer's or thinking about its possibility is a concern to nearly everyone today. Judah Ronch provides a thorough overview of how Alzheimer's affects victims and families, counseling approaches, the feelings counselors develop, and most importantly, ways to empower the helpers such as counselors or nurses who may at first become bewildered and disheartened when thinking about working with a disease that is progressively degenerative and always fatal. Practical approaches are stressed through many compassionate examples. One of the most creative chapters explains how to understand issues of separation and loss that occur in an ongoing way, affecting everyone in the family. While the book is oriented toward the general counselor and reader, a specialized section on diagnosis and assessment is presented in the appendix for readers desiring a more specialized outlook. Whether a social worker or a family member, a professional caregiver or simply a friend, anyone who deals with the painful consequences of Alzheimer's will benefit from this exceptionally helpful, and hopeful, volume.

Throughout the book Judah Ronch establishes his authority and expertise by writing about many of the things he has learned through thousands of hours of direct experience with victims of Alzheimer's and their families.

William Van Ornum, Ph.D.
Marist College
Poughkeepsie, New York

Preface

My own fascination with cognitive dysfunction and the dementias began with a demonstration of how the cognitively impaired think, which I witnessed at the Miami Jewish Home and Hospital for the Aged in September 1975. I was just beginning my first professional position in gerontology, and was interested to note that by analyzing the "incorrect response" or errors made by dementia patients, it was possible to understand their thought processes better. There were a small number of people studying cognitive impairment in the aging then, and even fewer working on ways of treating the devastation caused by dementing disorders.

Things have evolved since 1975 in the field of geriatrics and dementia care, and we have become a society thirsting for knowledge about the late-life dementia which may await so many of us. Care-givers of all kinds are increasingly having to do—as I did on that first job—learn as much and as quickly as possible as the need to counsel both Alzheimer's-disease victims and their families presents itself. Helpers are doing this in the many settings where older people and their relatives receive assistance of various kinds.

My experience as a psychologist, educator, program developer, and institutional consultant has shown me that all care-givers can indeed function as counselors to Alzheimer's victims and their families if properly trained. Staff can learn to hear "the question within the question," and how to respond in a manner that facilitates communication, comfort, and adaptive behavioral change. Such learning is possible when education is aimed at replacing labels with knowledge. Through this process, the "inappropriate" behavior of the demented elderly person comes to be seen as a consequence of neurological disease, and not as willful, childish, stubborn behavior that can be successfully eliminated by coercion, enough firmness, or appeals to a sense of shame or propriety. As a result of such training and education, staff and family intervention efforts are able to evolve from a combative, control-oriented interaction to one based on counseling and negotiation.

I have also seen how the "fear of senility" encourages judgmental, angry, phobic, and irrational "blaming the victim" responses on the part of well-intentioned family or professional care-givers, and in the nondemented elderly. Distance of a physical or psychological nature is so often put between "them," the demented Alzheimer's victims, and "us," the young, middle-aged or aging persons, as a barrier because of fear that this "senility" is contagious. This is an oft-repeated case of "gerontophobic" behavior, which can be readily eliminated when knowledge is put where labels (and moral judgments) had been. In this sense, this book will help persons become counselors *to themselves* through factual and affective education about Alzheimer's disease.

Reading this book will not eliminate the tragedy of Alzheimer's disease, or the disruption in people's lives (perhaps yours or someone you know) that this disease brings. I hope it will provide you with practical information so that you can proceed with your work, care for an afflicted relative or friend, or help someone who is coping with the constant stress of this disorder. Our desire as human beings is to "do the right thing," which in cases of Alzheimer's disease can appear to be an impossible goal. I hope that reading this book will help you to find "the right thing" to do.

You won't always get to do what you *want* to do, and "the right thing" may be something as difficult as doing nothing. When dealing with Alzheimer's disease, a good day feels like a constant series of compromises. On a bad day you're feeling overwhelmed, powerless, angry, guilty, or devastated.

I hope that some of the ideas in this book will sound like things you've thought or said to yourself, or that you will recognize a situation, outcome, dialogue, or description as familiar. Having your feelings or experience confirmed is one of the major therapeutic aspects of counseling, and feeling less alone is a most helpful thing to do when trying to contend with Alzheimer's disease.

The identities of the people written about in this book have been carefully disguised in accordance with professional standards of confidentiality and in keeping with their rights to privileged communication with the author. In some descriptions, however, true facts about these persons or about their symptoms have been retained to provide authenticity or preserve the illustrative value provided by that particular case example.

Acknowledgments

This book could not have been written without the help, support, and commitment of a number of very talented people. Whether by direct involvement with the manuscript or because they enriched my knowledge about pertinent issues of psychology, gerontology, and the dementias, these individuals all made contributions to the ideas and practices discussed in these pages.

I am very grateful to the patients and families I have met over the past fourteen years of clinical and consulting practice. They were the most effective teachers I could have had about what dementias do to people, and it is their experiences that I have attempted to convey to the reader through the ideas and examples found in the book. I hope that what they have endured will be both a lesson and a testament to us.

Drs. Rita D'Angelo, Virginia Sexton, Wagner Bridger, Sybil Barten, Vera John-Steiner, Vivian Horner, Henry Kellerman, and the late Herbert G. Birch all had a profound influence on my interest in psychology and human development. I am pleased to have this opportunity to acknowledge my indebtedness to them for all that they did by their lesson, example, and interest that made it possible for me to develop as a psychologist. Each of them made a unique contribution toward my understanding and appreciation of human development, behavioral organization, the role of temperament in development, and the relationships between language, thought, and culture as expressed in human behavior. This early experience provided me with a theoretical and investigatory framework which was fortunately at hand when I began work with the aging.

It was most fortuitous that I began my gerontological and geriatric career by learning from and working with Drs. Jack Skigen, Charles Beber, Norman Reichenberg, and the staff at the Douglas Gardens Outpatient Mental Health Center in Miami, Florida. It was at that pioneering, innovative place that Mr. Fred Hirt's and Dr. Jeffery Solomon's eagerness to develop professionals newly arrived to the field of aging and mental health helped me to establish myself in a field which has brought many personal and professional satisfactions. I am grateful for the collegiality, knowledge, and orientation to gerontology I experienced at Douglas Gardens and its parent institution, the Miami Jewish Home and Hospital for the Aged.

My involvement with dementia victims and their families continued at the Fishkill Health Related Center in Beacon, New York, where Mr. Lynn Kasin, the administrator, was eager to become involved in attempts at innovative care of the demented. His enthusiasm, commitment, and awareness of the magnitude of the change he was about to undertake as he sought to develop more effective care for the demented residents of his facility led to the establishment of a special care unit and a specially trained staff. For the past five years his and the staff's commitment and enthusiasm have allowed a care environment and training program to develop that has led to many of the notions and interventions I have described herein. I am pleased to acknowledge their many contributions, and to thank all of them for their willingness to experiment and to take an active role in the development of new approaches in dementia care. I have also been most fortunate to have Dr. S. Robert Watsky as a colleague both at Fishkill Health Related Center and in my private practice. His good humor and genuine commitment to interdisciplinary intervention has contributed significantly to the work I have been able to do.

It has been my pleasure to know and learn from Dr. Raymond Vickers, a superb geriatrician and psychiatrist, and a most gifted teacher. His informal tutorials about diagnostic and treatment issues in dementia care, and his constant willingness to be helpful when I was unclear about how to proceed in a given situation have made a major contribution to my thinking about Alzheimer's and other dementias.

I wish to thank Bill Van Ornum, who as editor of the series of which this book is one part suggested that I write this volume, and was always helpful and available each step of the way as it was written. His considerable skills as an author, psychologist, and editor helped to make the book more clear, precise, and comprehensive. Patricia Kane has my undying gratitude for grappling with my handwritten manuscript and turning it into a finished text. Her steadfast dedication and contributions to the content of the book based on her own professional experiences as a nurse made her a key to this book's completion. I hope that my endless thankfulness in some way compensates for the temporary (but considerable) impossibility of reading my handwriting. In this regard I wish to thank Michelle Kane for assisting her mother in this arduous task.

My final thanks go to Robin Doremus, RN, Director of Health Services at Fishkill Health Related Center, and the original clinical coordinator of the special care unit for dementia at that facility. Her considerable skills and the culture of care she promoted (then as now) have allowed for the empowering of the residents and staff so that all might function at the highest level. Many of the approaches to problem behaviors I discuss herein were developed by her, and I thank her for sharing them with all of us who work with her. She was a major source of assistance and support in the realization of this book with regard to both the clinical content and communicative precision of the manuscript. Without her personal and professional dedication, this book could not have been written.

This disease is a maniac. . . . I hate this disease.
—M. Roach

In the midst of neural devastation, there is much we can do.
—A. R. Luria

1

The Impact of Alzheimer's Disease on the Victim

Alzheimer's disease happens to people, not just to their brains. We may have to remind ourselves to keep this in mind in light of the emphasis on cognition and neurology given in much of the current literature on Alzheimer's and related disorders. It is probably not the case that the person experiencing the disease has been purposely ignored, but rather that we are currently more skilled in studying brain cells and investigating cognitive deficits than we are in capturing, defining, and categorizing the nature of what makes each person unique. Our challenge, nevertheless, is to do something on that order as best we can, since Alzheimer's disease causes, above all, the loss of the very essence that helps make the victim a unique "self" among others. Gone are memories of life's experiences and the capacity to behave in a thoughtful, reflective, "civilized" way that enables the person to recognize a congruence with who they are and who they have been.

An example of this process is the case of Mrs. Molly Gruber, a former storekeeper in a small town. By her mideighties her cognition had become so impaired that her family chose to place her in a skilled-nursing facility. Like many other people at this facility, Molly was ambulatory and otherwise healthy but markedly confused. Had she stayed at home, she would have been in physical danger. Her family was unable to provide twenty-four-hour care. Not long after being admitted, Molly began to wander in and out of other residents' rooms in the nursing home. She was brought to my attention because her constant searching through others' belongings (rummaging through their rooms, chests of drawers, closets, etc.) was making residents and staff alike feel very angry.

Part of Mrs. Gruber's problem became evident to me when I began to interview her—or at least tried to; her answers to my questions were a string of incomprehensible English words. Her medical chart indicated that she spoke two languages in addition to (the now unretrievable) English, so we conversed in the one other language we shared, a language she learned as a child (as had I). While no better oriented to time, place, or person when tested in her primary language, she was more relevant and expressive, and was able to speak with feeling and insight. (Her linguistic skills were not adapted in the nursing home since nobody else there spoke her language. Molly was in effect functionally aphasic of expressive language because nobody could understand.)

> COUNSELOR: Molly, I understand that you walk around this place all day, and go into other people's rooms. The nurses say that you look through other people's closets and drawers. Can you tell me why you do this?
>
> MRS. GRUBER: I look for Molly and I can't find her. I used to be able to read and enjoy myself, and I'd discuss what I had read with other people. But now I read and don't remember. That's not me, not the real Molly. So I walk around looking for Molly, but she's nowhere to be found.

The important insight Mrs. Gruber provides in this profound expression of what her dementia is like is that the goal of her behavior is to find HERSELF. She is looking for evidence that she had been somewhere in the past. Her searching through other people's belongings is an attempt at self-orientation. Through the search process, she had hoped to find objects she recognized as her own, stimuli that would trigger memories of a familiar, comforting past that now eluded her. Molly looked for traces of her impact on this new place (the nursing home) and, because she couldn't recognize herself anymore since she was unable *to do* what made her "the real Molly," she constantly searched the home trying to locate her.

Molly's eloquent description of the subjective puzzle that made up her daily life speaks of the need for counselors to take on the task of helping each victim find him- or herself. This task requires that we understand how these persons might be feeling in addition to how they think or what the level of their dysfunction is.

Loss of self is also expressed by persons with dementia who can no longer describe their predicament in the first person. Such expressions are sometimes communicated by descriptions of the plight of an "alter ego" who is really a projection of the self as it was during some period in the past. Ninety-year-old Miss Lipton, moderately impaired by Alzheimer's disease, wrote the following note and handed it to people who came to her home.

> Friends and relatives
> Hunting for a lost girl who has
> not been seen or recognized since
> yesterday, March fifth, by her peers,
> is leaving her identity and present plight
> unknown and unidentified and
> possibly in desperate need. Will you kindly
> stop and see if you can recall either the
> appearance or knowledge of such a young
> woman, and at once lend any possible
> information or assistance in locating or
> helping this missing person.

Phases of Change in Dementia

The loss of self each patient experiences will be of a unique nature even though patients may share similar patterns of cognitive disability. This consideration is almost self-evident as each person, each ego or "self," is an individual and will therefore undergo the loss of self-components that are individually developed, lifelong parts of daily physical, psychological, social, and biological functioning. The patient's experience will be in large part determined by how far he/she has come along physical, and emotional, development lines[1] and therefore which traits, relationships, skills, talents, and other characteristic components of his/her life will erode as dementia progresses and dematerializes the self. Dementia also requires that the patient (and his/her relatives) contend with developmental tasks already attained as well as those that will never occur.

Some of the developmental tasks in middle and late adulthood include:

Forties through Fifties

Middle-age body, physical changes, illness, body image.
Attitudes toward time.
Illness and death of contemporaries, parents.

Middle-age sex drive, activity, intimacy.
Relationship to spouse, partner.
Relationship to adult children, grandchildren.
Interaction with aging parents.
Friendship.
Resonance with friends of all ages.
Position of work, play.
Role as mentor.
Creativity.
Attitude toward money re: present, retirement, family, society.
Attitude toward and position in society.

Sixties and Beyond

Maintenance of body integrity.
Reaction to physical infirmity, impairment.
Attitude toward personal death.
Reaction to death of spouse, friends.
Reversal of roles with children, grandchildren.
Companionship vs. isolation and loneliness.
Role of sexual activity.
Retirement, use of time, continuance of meaningful work play.
Financial planning—attitudes toward self-care, surviving family members, society.[2]
(For a further discussion, see chapter 2.)

These tasks, or the psychosocial issues that must be successfully coped with if adult development is to proceed normally within a given cultural context, are the thematic components of middle age and later life's psychological work.

In Erik Erikson's terms, the achievement of generativity in later life (his seventh stage of man) is signaled by the unification of the person's personal, creative, ideational, and community lives when the person's productive life has assured that the individual's hopes, virtues, and wisdom will continue in the next generation.[3] The sense of failure to have achieved generativity is felt as feelings of self-absorption and stagnation. Progress toward the achievement of psychosocial growth along the developmental lines outlined above (as well as in earlier years of development) is the vehicle by which generativity is reached. In the final stage of life, the individual struggles to achieve integrity by having accepted his/her own and mankind's collective life cycles as something that by necessity permitted no substitutions.[4] It also means accepting responsibility for what happened during one's own life as one's own.[5] If it is acquired, a sense of integrity provides a successful solution to an opposing sense of despair and disgust . . . and of fear of death as the end to an unfulfilled life.[6] As the patient loses a clear awareness of the dimensions involved in his/her "categorical self"[7] during the course of Alzheimer's and other dementias, he/she drifts further away from a vantage point in the life cycle where a sense of generativity and/or integrity may be achieved.

This loss of self threatens the patient with unavoidable feelings of stagnation and despair. Early intervention to provide emotional support, particularly with life-review therapy[8] may be able to ameliorate some of these negative outcomes, though cognitive limitations may prevent the achievement or maintenance of sustained feelings of generativity or integrity. These are feelings that one gains gradually, however, and are not "all or nothing" achievements. This allows counseling efforts to produce some, albeit at times temporary, relief that may have a residual emotional impact on the patient and thereby provide comfort as cognition declines.

As the self is lost, the care-giving environment may be able to provide opportunities for restitution, which may enable the patient to feel more positive about the components of "categorical self" that remain. Patients who have available the people, objects, and emotional "supplies" matched to and congruent with their needs at all levels will have a greater opportunity to maintain their sense of self in spite of receding capacities and fading opportunities to experience all dimensions of the "categorical self."

The opportunity (not the requirement) to be with others can provide a chance for the patient to grow, to become, to enjoy— to "flourish."[9] Care providers in congregate (residential or outpatient) settings report that the opportunity to be with others and share the self in spite of significant cognitive impairment enables friendships to develop that utilize aspects of the "categorical self" (friend, companion, seductress, care-giver, coworker, comedian, audience, dancer, etc.) beyond those typically utilized in the home with the family. Relatives may at times experience feelings of guilt, jealousy, or confusion about why the patient did not act in this particular way while at home. Counselors or other care-givers can intervene by explaining the patient's enhanced adaptive ability in the program's environment that is structured to eliminate those aspects of adaptation the patient cannot achieve, and how different parts of the "categorical self" find expression in different environments. People who were not very social or who appeared depressed and withdrawn at home may become quite outgoing in a program environment designed for their care that is congruent with their skills and encourages enhanced expression of their "categorical selves" for as long as possible.

It is probably safe to say that a feeling of loss of control is common to dementia victims, a feeling that may be expressed verbally or behaviorally, such as by the intensification of defenses or by "acting up." The formulation of Cohen and others[10] provides us with an excellent basis from which to understand and discuss the evolution of subjective emotional reactions to the disorder. In so doing it also orients us toward the way to focus interventions at each phase, and realize that "not every individual with dementia experiences the phases in (this) order."[11] The psychologic phases may be overlapping or concurrent. These phases are guidelines rather than fixed immutable steps in a progression of change.

Phase One: Recognition and Concern

This phase starts prior to an actual diagnosis, when some cognitive change has been noted by patients and family members. These changes are frequently dismissed with "what do you expect at my age?" or as transient reactions to stress or life problems. Since the alterations in cognition are very subtle at the outset, it is both easy to deny their importance and difficult to identify a clear, consistent pattern of impairment. These changes ultimately become severe enough to be recognizable as those described in Phase One Dementia (see appendix A). This phase has been called "Recognition and Concern," because during this period of the disorder the dementia patient and family inevitably become aware of the serious change in the patient's behavior and are concerned about how to proceed. The patient may feel and/or verbalize things like "Something is wrong, I think I'm losing my mind" or "Am I crazy?" This latter question is usually an unarticulated though omnipresent one in the minds of most early-stage dementia victims, especially those in the current cohorts of aging persons. They remember that dementia was, in the past, treated as "insanity," and frequently led to involuntary institutionalization of patients in state psychiatric hospitals. Feelings such as these can make counseling difficult, especially if the reaction of the patients is fueled by the anxiety they feel about what will become of them, and by the anger and suspiciousness that may develop as they try to maintain their self-esteem, as in the case of Mrs. Brown (see Appendix A). Confusion and fear are only heightened if patients and their families are told, "It's only senility" or "This is normal at your mother's age."

Intervention

During this phase, it is important that the patient and his/her family find qualified professional help in order to enable them to obtain an explanation of why these changes have occurred (diagnosis). They should also seek aid in coping with the emotional reactions that accompany this stressful and frightening period in a family's life.

Phase Two: Denial/Relief

Some patients and families express denial, and steadfastly maintain that they haven't got any disorder—just "old age." Others have some mixed reactions, expressing a feeling that they are relieved to know they have a specific disease and that they are not insane, but they are upset by the news of what disease they have. They feel relief also at the prospect of not having to "cover up" for family and friends. Patients will occasionally express their ambivalence by strongly asserting both reactions, saying at one time: "Not me!" and at others: "I'm relieved to know that I'm not making this up or that I'm not crazy."

Intervention

Awareness of individual differences in the ability to cope is of paramount importance in this phase for anyone who wishes to provide assistance. Professionals must be honest and straightforward without overwhelming their patients in an attempt to "break through" their denial or resistance about accepting the bad news of the diagnosis.

The patient should be informed about the nature of the disease, what the future may hold, and the availability of family, friends, and professionals willing to help. It may require numerous counseling sessions to achieve some closure about these issues, since the patient's cognitive impairments, personality, support system, and the availability of competent helping professionals will all influence how long it takes for the person to adapt in this phase. Family, friends, neighbors, employers, and other important persons in the patient's social network should also be informed about the nature of the problem. The earlier in the progression of the disease the patient is told, the more easily can his/her intact cognitive abilities be utilized to accept the reality of the condition and the more readily can he/she be involved in planning for the future. The work of the counselor in this phase is like assembling a jigsaw puzzle that portrays the (unpleasant) new realities awaiting the patient and their family/caregivers. It must be done in small pieces, according to the tolerance of victim and family members so that the shock to the person's ego and the family system can be assimilated. Attempts to flood the family with reality through the use of aggressive confrontation are likely to heighten resistance and push them away from getting further help in the future.

Phase Three: "Why Me?"

"Why Me?," "What will happen to me?" are two common inquiries that occur in the process of assimilating the reality of the disease into the lives of its victims. The questions indicate the beginning of emotional upheaval and the point of transition to the planning phase. They indicate that the process of incorporating the fact of being demented into the patient's self-representation and into the world of his/her future has begun.

Patients exhibit shock, confusion, disorganization, guilt, sadness, rage, and other emotions in the period following the diagnosis. These emotions must be dealt with (often in counseling or supportive psychotherapy) if the patient is to become part of their treatment effort.

Dementia victims also may feel that they did something to cause the disease to befall them ("I must have gotten this because of something I did when I was in the service"), or may wonder "What did I do to deserve this?" They may also attribute their dementia to bad luck, a weak constitution, "God," or recall that a parent or grandparent had some similar problems late in life and wonder whether they inherited it.

Intervention

Counselors can be of great assistance if they help the patient accept the fact that he/she did not bring the disease about, and that no external forces are to blame. Successful adaptation to the disease can be facilitated by working with the patient to accept his/her feelings, to realize that he/she has had no control over the onset or existence of the disease, and that he/she nevertheless has some control over some aspects of life. These should be overtly discussed and negotiated with care-givers, so that the remaining strengths of the patient can be utilized in adaptation and maintained. If not, the patient will lose opportunities to behave competently and maintain self-esteem. Assuming that the presence of *some* impairment signifies total helplessness accelerates the patient's loss of self-esteem (and erodes the sense of who he/she is) and causes premature burdening of care-givers. It also encourages the occurrence of behavioral problems in the patient who has been prematurely defined as incompetent in all spheres, who will struggle to demonstrate to himself and others that he/she can still do things.

Many aged persons with dementia appear to be depressed or indeed display some of the symptoms of depression. Hopelessness, helplessness, and pessimism are not unnatural reactions to the knowledge that one has a progressive chronic disease. Allowing people with dementia to retain as much power and control over the important aspects of their lives as is safe is a significant way to forestall or minimize depression.

There is much work to be done during this phase, and proper counseling intervention can yield enormous benefits for the patient and family. A range of professionals might be needed at this phase, all of whose efforts can be enhanced by the use of appropriate counseling activities. Intervention is important at this juncture to assist the victim and the family with the "reorganization of the most important aspects of his or her personal life, relationships, and lifestyle."[12] Categories of intervention derived from Cohen et al and their discussion of helping activities include:

1. Assessment:
   A. Evaluate patient's level of functioning, intact capabilities, and disabilities.
   B. Evaluate resources family has available.
2. Education:
   A. Provide accurate information about Alzheimer's disease.
   B. Teach the family what they can expect their patient to do over time in light of current research and the personality of the patient.
   C. Provide the family with a list of resources they might require and make linkages for them with workers at each resource or service provider.
   D. Teach good communication skills to the family and friends (and other service providers) so that relationships may be maintained and improved.
3. Counsel:
   A. Discuss and explore the patient's and family member's feelings to facilitate acceptance of the disorder and understanding of everyone's (right to an) emotional reaction.
   B. Prevent or minimize depression by working with the patient and family towards developing a set of realistic expectations that can serve as guidelines for specific activities and limits that each person, patient included, can be expected to do as the disease progresses.
   C. Encourage the patient and family members to become involved in support and/or therapeutic groups so that they might feel less alone.

Phase Four: Coping

This phase entails adjusting to the changes that occur in the patient's functional ability while providing opportunities for the patient to flourish. Numerous endings must be generated to complete the sentence "In order to function I must..." It is not enough to "keep the patient busy," as this produces coping at a minimal level of competency and feelings of demoralization or depression in a demented person just as it would with someone with intact cognition. As Molly Gruber implied earlier in this chapter, a day well spent is a day when she can do the things she considers to be indicative of who she is as a person. In that spirit, the activities of this phase should be oriented toward helping the patient perpetuate the "I" by doing those things in such a way that the person knows him/herself. Individual patterns of likes and dislikes, preferences for certain routines in self care, meals, outings, etc. are helpful guidelines with which to allow continuity of self identification in the midst of cognitive decline.

Patients should be asked what they think or how they feel about things, especially when plans are to be changed or routines altered. The patient's ability to state his/her needs or desires can be brought to bear on many situations in order to facilitate or maximize—though certainly not guarantee—cooperation. Care-givers run the risk of provoking anger, withdrawal, or regression if they adopt a paternalistic posture and assume that they always know what is best for the patient. By the same token, our attitudes about the symptoms of the dementia or the disorder itself are not necessarily those of the patient. The latter can be elicited and explored in a counseling interaction to help with behavior problems.

As persons with dementia experience the loss of more and more skills, they should be helped to maintain their dignity by being encouraged to maintain maximum possible autonomy with safety. A person feels less capable of coping if he/she is constantly being told that his/her decisions are wrong or that "you should know better." Issues over which to disagree should involve matters crucial to the well-being of the patient and not issues of simple aesthetics or personal choice. For example, the color of the pants a person chooses to put on is not important, but whether or not pants (shirt, dress, skirt, etc.) are worn when going outdoors or when people are in the home are issues worthy of intervention.

Intervention

Counseling in this phase involves assisting the care-givers with the practical plans of everyday living and facilitating service linkages to promote integration, evaluation, and future planning of resources. In this phase especially a good deal of counseling may be required as regards to: (1) coping with the patient's changing levels of capability, (2) feelings about surrendering autonomy and control to care-givers; and (3) renegotiating family "contracts" about who will do what for the patient and the patient's feelings about who shall and should give care. Counseling may also be necessary to discuss alternatives to home-based care if the community does not offer appropriate and/or sufficient services to make living at home a safe and viable option for the demented person as disabilities increase. Emotion-laden topics such as nursing-home placement, coping with hospitalization, and potential behavior problems while hospitalized are frequent topics of counseling intervention.

Phase Five: Maturation

"Living one day at a time until I die" is one way to describe how patients with dementia live. Their lives have been called "the ultimate existential existence, living each day as if it were the only one."[13] Not all demented patients are able to achieve maturation due to the impact of their cognitive losses.[14] Maturation is achieved in instances where a special bond exists between patient and caregiver whether the latter is a spouse, a child, a friend, or a paid worker. This bond leads the patient (and not incidentally the caregiver) to feel worthwhile, cared for and cared about, and to experience a sense of mastery over some things despite the severe debilitation that has by this point in the dementia imposed major limitations on the patient's physical, cognitive, and psychosocial functioning.

Intervention

Maturation can be achieved in the home-care or institutional setting, so long as there is consistent, intimate, personal care available. Counselors should continue to focus on the patients active involvement in his/her own life, his/her need for self-determination and competency through mastery of even minor obstacles. The assessment of need for services and provision of linkage to resources should continue simultaneously. Ongoing support for the patient and family, as well as the opportunity to help and be helped by others through peer support groups or telephone support, are advisable for the duration of this and earlier phases.

During this phase, patients can be made to feel less anxious if they are part of something more continuous than their own fragmented experience. For them, as for young infants, affective bonds are central to the potential for feelings of continuity. While dementia patients may not remember people's names, they apparently retain emotional afterimages for long-enough intervals to develop feelings of trust and security about certain care-givers. Angry interactions, on the other hand, can leave a residue of fear and mistrust for the patient. He/she may react with anger the next time a care-giver is encountered. Informal counseling during care routines and daily activities are a way of helping the patient process his/her feelings. Putting feelings into words for people who cannot articulate their emotions, and having these expressions validated is a very useful and therapeutic activity through which care-givers can assist the patient in the maturation process. Professional counselors who are experts in this field but who do not work with the patient on a day-to-day basis can provide supervisory consultation to direct care staff about how to do this while not interposing their own feelings in the maturation process.

Phase Six: Separation from Self

"This is a stage that no patient has ever been able to express," say Cohen et al,[15] but it is nevertheless a stage where we can observe that a great deal is happening to the patient. By this time the patient is able to receive information to a far greater extent than he/she can express it, and cannot play an active role in his/her life or environment. The total physical dependency experienced by the patient makes his/her degree of comfort a major area of experience. As the person approaches death, comfort and security become the focus of the family, even as they begin to deal with their ambivalent feelings around the loss of their loved one who will be liberated from suffering by death.

Intervention

Verbal and tactile messages of concern, support, reassurance, and love are the tools available to all care-givers as they counsel the person in this final phase. Counseling can impact and/or reinforce a sense of dignity in the midst of the multiple indignities of this disease, through a steadfast maintenance of contact with the humanness of the patient.

This look at the patient's emotional responses to his/her dementia and the ensuing alterations of interpersonal relationships is intended to accomplish a number of objectives. First, it hopefully will illustrate the point that people do not become progressively demented without having some emotional reaction. Though many families or care-givers express feeling like "Sam could do better if he tried, he's just being lazy," or "Minerva just likes the attention she gets when she has things done for her," these are not always incorrect or signs of denial of the illness. They may be astute analysis of the role that the patient's personality is playing in the adaptive picture.

The second point to be made is that an individual's lifelong personality traits are a guide to, but not a totally accurate prediction of, how they will respond to the increased anxiety, loss of control, and loss of self-esteem that go along with watching one's mind dissolve. If the person never communicated his/her feelings easily prior to becoming demented regular, insightful self-expression is not likely to occur. A person who characteristically has been aggressive may try to compensate for feeling as if he/she is losing control by becoming more aggressive, and a rigid, compulsive person may become more rigid.

A good history from an accurate, reliable informant will help the counselor put the personality changes, manifestations of increased anxiety, and coping style demonstrated by the patient into perspective. It is, in addition, a useful reference point for the family and care-givers who can help by supporting available strengths during care-giving, allowing them to abandon fantasies that their patient, spouse, or parent will suddenly and magically change in dramatic fashion if only dealt with in the "correct" way. Realistic goals for care can be more easily set and, hopefully, more readily attained if the patient's individual history is factored into care planning and execution. Such goal setting leaves patients and family members/care-givers feeling more competent and less angry. These issues provide a counseling intervention for the duration of the illness.

Finally, to the extent that the Alzheimer's patient lives in a social world composed of friends, family, coworkers, and acquaintances, the disease has many victims. The next chapter will look into the impact of Alzheimer's disease on the family and friends of the patients—the additional victims of the disease.

2

Separation and Loss in Alzheimer's Disease: The Impact on the Family

Introduction

"Make the diagnosis and treat the family" was the axiomatic advice that used to be given to professionals working with suspected cases of Alzheimer's disease and related disorders. It was not so long ago (within the last decade) that the family of the patient received the ongoing treatment since it was believed that nothing could be done for the patient anyway. Recent innovations[1] in the care of dementia victims have demonstrated the undue pessimism of the "treat only the family" approach, but the family remains the major target of the bulk of care-giving interventions in Alzheimer's disease. Family members provide most of the care to patients and can derive long-range benefit from intervention. They also require immediate, short-term relief from the stresses of care-giving and all the strain of coping with the illness(es). Books like *The Thirty-six Hour Day*,[2] *The Loss of Self*,[3] and *Alzheimer's Disease: A Guide for Families*[4] are three of the more outstanding resources offered to help families cope with the physical and emotional toll of caring for a demented person. Their comprehensive coverage of these topics makes them required reading for family care-givers and counselors who will work with families. In addition, the accessibility of these books and the clarity of their message makes it possible for the reader to consult them directly in order to obtain the full undiluted flavor of their contributions. Reading those (or related) works will give the professional a great deal of insight into what the family/care-giver faces, and will add invaluable knowledge and perspective to the counseling and other assistance he/she can provide family members.

This discussion will focus on the emotional turmoil left in the wake of the damage caused when Alzheimer's disease and related dementias loot the mind and break the heart.[5] A counselor may be asked to go beyond the stage of appraisal, information, and referral when helping a family, and proceed to assist that family as it copes with the emotionally draining process that occurs simultaneous with care giving—enduring the grief process during the "funeral that never ends."[6]

A Unique Pattern of Losses

Alzheimer's disease and other dementias make numerous demands on the victims and their family members. These are the demands of actual care giving and bearing psychological and physical burdens,[7] and the work that must be done to cope with the impact of a relationship in transition. As the disabilities of the patient require that formerly intact capacities be assumed by another, the nature of the interpersonal bond between patient and the family undergoes significant modifications. Family members and the patient must contend with the impact of an evolution of role changes, alterations in habitual modes of relating to each other on both emotional and intellectual bases, as well as revised expectations of future plans.

Progressive dementias require that patients and family members endure an ongoing process whereby each experience separation and loss of the other. They experience an ever-widening gap between "what is" and "what used to be." They watch helplessly as "what could have been" (the real and unrealistic fantasies and expectations about the future) becomes "what will never be." Unlike other chronic illnesses that do not affect mentation, progressive dementias prevent the patient from continuing to be an ongoing, active partner in the mutual process of letting go. Though the experience of separation and loss is a mutual complementary process shared by the patient and family members, only the latter maintain the potential to be consciously aware of, reflect about, and express their feelings. But the behavior of dementia patients demonstrates that they are also experiencing a process of separation and loss, though their expressions of this experience are perhaps of a different nature. Molly (chapter 1) looks for "herself," other patients look for their mothers or search for a home that is missing. Mrs. Lipton (chapter 1) gives notes to visitors asking whether anyone has seen a lost girl or knows anything about this "missing person." In early stages of dementia, patients can express feelings to the spouse that they "soon won't know anything and I'll be happy. You're the one I feel sorry for."[8] Patients' reaction to separation and loss at all levels of dementia seem to be at variance with more conservative assessments of the patients' ability to grieve losses.[9]

There is a unique quality to the experience of separation and loss in Alzheimer's disease owing to the series of multiple, concatenated, serial losses caused by the dementia on the patient and significant others. The loss of the "self" that the patient experiences and the loss of the patient by loved ones both conform to this pattern that can be described as "canonical" in nature. This term is used to emphasize the nature of the pattern of losses like a canon in music, a pattern where a melody begins and is repeated from the beginning while the initial melody line continues. It is difficult to describe and appreciate the nature of this process if you haven't gone through it. Marion Roach, the daughter of an Alzheimer's disease victim has written:

> It goes on and on, and just when we can't stand another phase, we don't have to, because it's succeeded by another one—a worse phase, a more outrageous phase, a quieter phase, a sloppier phase, a more confused phase, a phase of hushed panic—seen in the eyes of the victim, seen by us.[10]

Simply put, the person with progressive dementia (Alzheimer's or any other) appears to be "dissolving," missing. "We witness ghostly transformations, people who were loving and loved become morbid distortions of themselves. What is gone is personhood."[11] As the person "dissolves," the family member can begin to feel as Marion Roach did, that "Alzheimer's is a disease of separation"[12] in which one begins to separate from loved ones. "As when I first went away from home to sleep overnight at a friend's house, or first went off to camp, or first went to college at eighteen, I have had to learn again about separation,"[13] says Roach. In contrast to these separations, however, the separations of Alzheimer's disease do not promise reunion as a reward for patience. Roach's developmentally timely separations from her family were steps along the road from dependency toward autonomy. She would return to her family more mature, more autonomous, less dependent on them, closer to responsible adulthood. The separation from her mother brought on by Alzheimer's disease was forced upon her and promised no reunion, only more losses. Her transition from autonomous young adult to care-giving, dependable daughter is described in eloquent terms[14] and illustrates her return to a dependency relationship with her mother, though this time her mother, not she, was the partner in need of loving emotional and physical nurturance.

A key difficulty experienced by family members, especially those who are care-givers, is that they are prevented from experiencing the normal grieving process by which people come to terms with losses. Grief is an emotional response to loss, which, in the case of a death, can be overwhelming at first and become less intense with time. In a chronic illness however "just when you think you have adjusted, the person may change and you will go through the grieving experience again."[15] The feelings of sadness, anger, fatigue, guilt, and despair that accompany grief are restimulated each time another element vanishes that makes the patient a person.

The loss of the person in bits and pieces while he/she is physically there inspires feelings such as these:

> Sometimes I feel like I have a big hole in my stomach. It's open and empty and so painful. It aches and begs to be filled with a touch, some sign of understanding, something that will somehow bond Ray and me again.... He doesn't know that I hurt and can't make the emptiness and loneliness go away. And yet he is physically there.[16] I know I lost Ray long before he actually died. I lost the part of him that made him the man I found so satisfying. We complimented each other. As he deteriorated, we lost that.[17]

As the patient loses the parts of him/herself that formed the boundaries and internal structures by which the person experienced "wholeness" an internal process takes place. In a cruel, endlessly teasing way, this process of disappearing before one's own eyes must be understood and coped with as the intellectual tools by which this might have been done become unavailable. Feelings of anxiety and sadness cannot always be adequately prevented from overwhelming the patient with an almost-incomprehensible flood of confusion, fright, and frustration. The patient knows that something is happening, that there are "big holes"[18] where knowledge used to be, and feels that there are "rules to things and I just don't know how to do it"[19] but isn't able to defend against feelings of anxiety brought on by such a realization. As the person vanishes, so too do his/her barriers to fear and insecurity. The psychological work necessary to grieve such a "loss of self" and come to terms with dying[20] cannot be completed because the intellectual mechanisms necessary for insight, introspection, and closure break down. Patients are therefore predisposed toward feelings of despair[21] as they become less capable of coming to terms with what is happening to them.

Patients' feelings about this process are sometimes evident to family members/care-givers because they are verbalized; such as when Mr. Garfman tells a nurse, "I am looking for me but I really don't know where I am." They can also be understood on an intuitive basis by insightful relatives/care-givers who note the sense of personal alienation, withdrawal, and aura of being lost that characterizes many patients. Relatives may feel guilt, inadequacy, anger, sadness, and even fear for their own futures as they comprehend the meaning of the patient's behavior. The family member/care-giver bears the unenviable burden of having to think for both parties in this separation process, and must try to cope with his/her own feelings as they effect the relationship with the patient.

Case Example

Mrs. Knight is the daughter-in-law of an Alzheimer's patient and the mother of a three-year-old child born after the Knights were past forty years of age. She expressed a great ambivalence about visiting her mother-in-law after she became aware of her guilt feelings toward her own child. "I asked myself, what have we done to her? Did we saddle our daughter with the responsibility of caring for us if we became confused just as she's at the point of starting her own life as an adult?"

Grief and Alzheimer's Disease

As was stated above, grieving the many losses of Alzheimer's disease and other dementias follows a pattern that is probably unique among illness. Society's support for this process is often found to be lacking by the grieving family because the patient doesn't "look sick," is still physically present, and the visible loss of a person (to death) has not happened. This apparent lack of societal ceremony or mechanism to assist the grieving family is an added source of burden that intensifies their already very stressful "canonical grief."

Before we can pursue a discussion of the nature of the grief process in Alzheimer's disease, it is necessary to define grief's components. Wisocki and Averill[22] describe the four stages of normal grieving as:

1. *Shock*—a dazed sense of unreality that may last anywhere from hours to days. The person may feel numb or isolated from the world, a feeling that can continue into subsequent stages.
2. *Protest and Yearning*—the loss is recognized but not entirely accepted. Intense pain and a strong longing for the deceased occur. This is followed by *protest* over the loss, and *searching* for the lost person (through dreams or finding a sense of the person in familiar places). The bereaved person may become preoccupied with memories of the lost person and pay a great deal of attention to aspects of the environment associated with past pleasures they shared.
3. *Disorganization and Despair*—this is the most enduring and difficult phase and can last a year or more. The bereaved person feels bitter, may pine away after the deceased but without continuing attempts at "recovery." Apathy, withdrawal, loss of energy, despondency, and beginning signs of depression (appetite change, sleep disturbances, loss of libido, isolation, etc.) may occur. Conflicting emotions—e.g., anger and sadness, irritability, and guilt are experienced.
4. *Detachment, Reorganization, and Recovery*—as healing proceeds toward completion, the person begins to develop new ways of thinking about the world and establishes new relationships with a sense of purpose. Life can be enjoyed again, though the pain of loss may never subside completely.

When a person dies suddenly or after a brief illness, the process of grieving would normally be expected to follow the above description. A long-term chronic illness without cognitive impairment extends the process but permits the possibility of mutual disengagement prior to death between patient and loved ones. The patient can be helped to come to terms with dying as a process in the life cycle,[23] an activity that can bring solace to patient and family alike. Chronic dementing illnesses do not even afford the patient and family a chance at such consolation, and the relatives typically experience the process of losing the patient without having had an opportunity to say good-bye.[24]

The progressive disappearance of the dementia patient necessitates that the survivor(s) grieves the separation from and loss of all that was the person *while the person is still physically present to trigger memories of what is lost.* Doernberg writes, "I live with memories. The man I love is but a shell of himself. It's a tease. He is there, but not there. He is a member of our family, and yet not the same member of the family."[25] The outstanding characteristics of a person—friendliness, decisiveness, sense of humor, ability to make others feel secure, a giving nature—begin to fall away and as they do so they disassemble and transform previous role relationships. A wife goes from lover to care-giver,[26] a daughter from child to care-giver, as the person each knew is unable to perpetuate what he/she once was to the life of the others.

Impact on the Spouse

A spouse of a dementia patient experiences an unraveling of the intricate network of connections built up over the history of the relationship. The bridges between the two, felt to be present, by the dependable security and comfort they give, fade away. The loss of intellectual companionship, financial support, child-rearing efforts, nurturance, etc., combine with a loss of mutuality and emotional expression (yet the patient can show distress at seeing the care-giver spouse upset) to make the care-giving spouse feel as though he/she is spouseless but married. Their sexual relationship suffers and ceases to play any positive role as the demented spouse becomes sexually disinterested, overinterested, unable to remember how to make love, and/or catastrophically reactive.[27] The care-giving spouse may feel less sexual interest in the partner than before, either because the change in the patient has led to a changed perception of the patient (from lover to dependent) or because the grief process has led to a withdrawal of emotional energy from the demented spouse. The unimpaired spouse will also likely have to struggle with a loss of friends who are uncomfortable relating to a third person rather than to another couple as before.[28] One distressed seventy-seven-year-old woman who had recently agreed to nursing-home placement for her moderately demented husband lamented about the near total abandonment by "their" friends, and was hurt because none of them visited him in the nursing home. "I plead with them to visit him, and none of them call me to invite me over anymore. You'd think we have something contagious," she said.

The spouse of a dementia patient is unable to proceed through the grieving process to find emotional equilibrium because the losses discussed above happen in a relentless series. The newly perceived loss interrupts the grief over a previous one and the process begins anew over the next aspect of the person or spousal relationship that vanishes. Shock is perhaps short-lived as realities of care giving force the spouse to pay attention to the actual manifestations of the loss—e.g.; a need for more physical care, trouble expressing needs, increased disorientation, etc. The protest-and-searching phase appears to be the likeliest place where a care-giving spouse can become mired down as the patient is indeed constantly found in familiar places but is behaving in a totally unfamiliar way. The spouse ends up searching for the unimpaired person and protesting over the loss of that individual. This cycle can be repeated in a seemingly constant pattern until the patient is totally disabled and there is little left to provide fresh reminders to the spouse of the unimpaired individual. Doernberg describes her feelings in this way: "I feel like I'm in limbo. I can't look ahead, but it's too painful to stay where I am. I try to let go and I can't. I grieve so. I know it is over, and yet he is there to remind me of what is no longer."[29] This is an eloquent description of the disorganization and despair to which Wisocki and Averill[30] refer.

Spouses who think about picking up the pieces of their lives often feel conflict about such behavior. Here again they are prevented from doing normal grief work by the series of losses they continue to experience, yet they are unable to continue to live the life of a married person due to their spouse's disabilities. In the eyes of society they are a wife, but day-to-day realities challenge the usual definition of this role for them.

> I have a husband but not a husband. He is physically present and mentally alert for me to still consider him as a person who has feelings, thoughts, and is somewhat aware. But he does not provide anything for me. I don't know how to fill this void.[31]

Being neither "wife nor widow" creates a peculiar status for a spouse who likely will have to abandon vocational, professional, recreational, and other interests for the duration of care giving and thereby become socially isolated. He/she may feel the need to go out among others when the need for companionship and peer relations gets particularly strong, especially near the end of the dementing illness. Desires like these can produce feelings of guilt and fears of social rejection or censure by others, or feelings of awkwardness when out with other couples.

Perhaps the best way to clarify the foci for counseling around a spouse's loss is to describe the developmental context in which these losses take place. The literature on the tasks of adult development is not as comprehensive as is the child-development literature, and despite some notable exceptions[32] not much is available of a coherent theoretical or empirical nature to help clinicians who wish to place adult psychosocial phenomena into a developmental context. Colarusso and Nemiroff[33] have applied Freud's[34] concept of developmental lines to help us understand some of the tasks of adult and later-life development. These are particularly instructive if we wish to understand along which domains some of the losses occur as an adult separates from a cognitively impaired spouse. Outlined and discussed below are selected developmental lines taken from Colarusso and Nemiroff's[35] full discussion of this topic used to illustrate the nature of the content of separation and loss. A choice has been made to focus on middle (forty through sixty) and late (sixty and beyond) adulthood to enhance clarity and since the majority of spouses and patients will fall into these groups.

Intimacy, Love, and Sex

(Forties through Fifties)

- Increased recognition of the value of long-standing relationships.
- Redefunction of relationships to partner as children grow and leave.
- Ability to care for partner in face of illness, aging, physical retrogression.
- Capacity to share new activities, interests, and people.
- Continuation of active sex life.
- Acceptance of loss of procreative ability in women.

(Sixties through Seventies)

- Capacity to tolerate loss, death of partner, friends.
- Ability to form new sustaining ties with friends, children, grandchildren.
- Continuation of active sex life.

The Alzheimer's impaired individual is unable to play a normal part in the development of the spouse along this developmental line. The long-standing relationship that exists cannot be valued without at the same time painfully recognizing that it is in the process of being lost. Bittersweet memories occur as the unimpaired spouse remembers the past and how valuable the relationship has been while being forcibly separated from the relationship as it was. An undeniable awareness grows that the much-desired, long-standing relationship is not to be, and from this theoretical perspective, this developmental line will stop developing as will other dimensions that follow below. The relationship cannot be redefined as might be expected when children grow and leave, since a mutual, mature, balanced relationship marked by the pursuit of common goals "now that the children are gone" is not possible. Instead, the unimpaired spouse sees the spousal relationship redefined as caregiver and dependent while separating from the interdependent spousal roles once played by both partners. The ability to care for the partner in the face of illness and cognitive disability is challenged endlessly and becomes the entire focus of the intact partner's life. New interests, activities, and people cannot be shared as the patient's cognitive impairment precludes adapting to new situations, people, events, etc., and undermines his/her ability to adapt to what once had been enjoyable friendships, pursuit of interests, and routine activities. The spouse may not only *not* proceed without conflict along this dimension to develop new interests, etc., but is under constant pressure to suspend his/her life while serving as the primary care-giver. Only after the loss has been grieved—and protracted losses can produce extended grieving periods—can he/she pick up the pieces and resume an approximation of a "normal life." Continuing with an active sex life is also subject to the obvious difficulties discussed above.

It can be concluded that the forties-fifties are times when the unimpaired spouse sees many premature terminations of normal developmental tasks in the intimacy, love, and sex developmental line. This experience is likely to be felt at some level of awareness but perhaps not consciously perceived as a global, massive separation from one's own developmental destiny in this area. The impaired spouse is likewise deterred from continuing his/her developmental work, but is rendered unable to process, consider, and develop compensatory strategies for these events.

The Body

(Fifties through Sixties)

- Reaction to the experience of physical decline.
- Reactions to physical impairment, hearing or vision loss, diseases, etc.
- Ability to compensate for diminished physical energy, altering schedule, diet, sleep patterns, etc.
- Care of the body, regular exercises, appropriate health care.

(Seventies)

- Ability to remain active and outgoing in the face of frequent physical infirmity.
- Acceptance of permanent physical impairment and chronic illness.
- Continued exercise and care of the body vs. neglect.

The care-giving spouse is confronted with a paradox and the need to compromise developmental work. At a time when physical changes related to normal aging or due to illness(es) occur, the spouse is called upon to expend considerable energy and subject him/herself to the stress of physical and emotional overwork. It has become common to hear of care-giver spouses who become ill or die not long after the death or institutional placement of the demented spouse, apparently victims of their own dedication and truly victims of the spouse's dementia. Thus, normal development would have the unimpaired spouse do things and adjust to physical changes or illness by conserving physical capacity while using the body in such a way as to keep it strong. Being a care-giver to a demented spouse does not allow such a measured allocation of physical resources. Accepting physical changes (visual impairments, arthritis, cardiac conditions, etc.) is not as easily accomplished when one feels that somebody (e.g., the spouse) is not available to give assistance, and when these changes prevent the spouse from fulfilling responsibilities for the demented partner's care.

Time and Death

(Fifties through Sixties)

- Acceptance of the preciousness of time, leading to an increased interest in the quality of experience.
- Effect of personal vulnerability, illness, aging on thoughts of time and death.
- Effect of death of loved one.
- Continued interest in present and future vs. dwelling on the past.

(Seventies)

- Integrity vs. despair.
- Preparation for personal death.

This developmental line is the focus of a great deal of psychological work for the spouse. The patient is rendered unable to do the requisite work past the early stages of dementia, though the loss of self proceeds. Care-taking spouses realize all too well that time is both an ally and an enemy. The demented "person" living in the present is perpetually dematerializing; awareness of the preciousness of time promotes recognition by the unimpaired spouse that there is little time to enjoy what both have together. In Alzheimer's and other progressive dementias, time is experienced as the abductor, relentlessly taking as it passes the person who was there just before. But it proceeds not quickly enough for some spouses, who have come to terms with the inevitable loss of their husband/wife and wish for both selfish and altruistic reasons that the disappearance of their partner would come to a merciful end. Counselors are confronted with the family members' extended canonical grieving process, the ambivalence about time, and the care-giving spouse's needs to integrate thoughts about the death of his/her partner with the thoughts this stimulates regarding his/her own eventual death. These issues can come up repeatedly throughout the protracted grieving period as the temporary equilibrium achieved by the partner is upset by yet another loss which reopens this subject again as grief continues.

Relationships to Children

(Fifties through Sixties)

- Facilitation of adult children's development (financially, emotionally).
- Establishment of mature friendships with grown children.
- Acceptance of one's position in the older generation—grandparenthood.
- Relationships to grandchildren.

(Seventies)

- Continued facilitation of grown children's and grandchildren's development.
- Acceptance of reversal of roles, help, support from middle-aged children.

The complexion of relationships with one's children changes drastically when a parent has dementia. The cognitively impaired parent is essentially unable to achieve a lasting maturation along this developmental line, and may be prevented from attaining many personally significant milestones within dimensions along this line. The unimpaired spouse has his/her attention diverted, energies monopolized, resources eaten up, and role as a grandparent compromised by the demands of being a care-giver. Role reversals with children become apparent in some relationships earlier than they might have in development, particularly if the stress of care giving compromises the health of the cognitively intact spouse. (This subject will be discussed in greater detail later when the effect on adult children is explained.) Psychological development along this developmental line is clearly at risk for both spouses. But once again we can see that only the unimpaired partner will have to cope with the emotional stress of separating from what might have been and possibly losing what could have been a golden opportunity to develop relationships within the family that could have promoted better adaptation to old age.

Work

(Forties through Fifties)

- Continued development of skills and achievement.
- Acceptance of failure to reach certain goals.
- Choice of new or second career.
- Working for society, others.
- Use of power, position.

(Sixties through Seventies)

- Continued involvement in meaningful work and play.
- Attitude toward retirement.

Finances

(Forties through Fifties)

- Ability to use money for present pleasure.
- Planning for the future—insurance, savings, college for children, retirement.

(Sixties and Beyond)

- Adaptation to retirement income.
- Plans for money after ones own death, making a will, providing for spouse, children, community.

Play

(Forties, Fifties, and Beyond)

- Increased capacity for mental hobbies and play as ability for physical play diminishes.

- Effect of increased leisure on play; meaningful use of time vs. pleasureless activities.

The developmental lines of work, finances, and play have been presented together to reflect the intertwined effect Alzheimer's disease and related disorders have on the lives of the spouse and patients. There is a great deal of separation and loss in each of these areas that occurs in a cyclical pattern. That is, as the ability to work is reduced by the patient's impairment or the spouse's having to forego work in order to care for the patient, financial losses usually follow. Money earmarked for retirement, travel, pleasure, savings, college tuition for children, and one's estate is quickly used up paying for care and as a means of supporting the family when the income is interrupted. One spouse wondered how she would afford twenty thousand dollars a year to pay for an at-home caretaker (a rather modest sum in some geographical areas) and still have the money she needed for her two son's annual college tuitions.[36] Since many insurance plans will not pay for the kind of supervisory care dementia patients need, and others deny benefits for hospital stays because the condition is deemed either psychiatric (with limited coverage in most cases) or "untreatable," money disappears rapidly. The unimpaired spouse must cope with separation from both his/her financial resources as well as a financially secure future. Spouses must often leave the work force at an age when reentry becomes impractical. They are likely to be considered too old to be a good candidate for employment. Older couples face the problem of having been able to establish a financially secure base on pension income, only to see it eaten up by the costs of caring for an Alzheimer's or otherwise-demented spouse that are not covered by Medicare, Medicaid, or any other insurance program.

Counseling Considerations

The preceding discussion was included so that counselors may have a systematic approach with which to assess the impact of dementia on a spouse's growth and development as a human being. It is easy to be distracted from the fact that development continues throughout the life span, and that while the spouse copes with the daily chores of caring for a demented partner, his/her psychological development is significantly affected. A major consideration in counseling the spouse of a patient is to be concerned with the day-to-day practical care issues he/she experiences, and with the covert psychological and emotional processes that are happening as he/she tries to struggle with everyday life. The pattern of continuous loss and the resulting lack of opportunity to complete grieving for each loss, and the interruption and/or cessation of personal growth along the developmental lines discussed above can produce significant emotional difficulties in the intact spouse. Counseling can provide both short-term help and long-lasting benefit if the emotional needs and developmental opportunities of the intact spouse are considered as important and valued goals of intervention.

The concept of developmental lines has been presented in addition so that the counselor can utilize them as an organizing structure of perspective when obtaining a history, listening to a client, or preparing to offer feedback on how he/she sees the many problem areas in the spouse's life. Clients may find it helpful to have their many and often disorganized thoughts reflected back to them in a way that recognizes their needs (as opposed to the usual focus on the patient). They may also be encouraged to plan for and think about their lives in terms of reached, postponed, or canceled goals, or tasks to be done. In the midst of the stressful emotional reaction spouses often experience when a partner is impaired by dementia, it can be comforting to be helped when a systematic approach is offered. This does not have to be done formally, but can be accomplished by reflective listening and clarification about which developmental line the spouse is concerned.

Impact on Children of the Patient

The offspring of a dementia patient face a grieving process that is similar in dynamics to what the spouse experiences but differs in the particular qualities of role changes and relational dynamics that are inherent in parent-child relationships. Children of Alzheimer's and other dementia patients experience a drastic modification of what was "normal" as their parent becomes less able to remain independent. They must therefore grieve the loss of a parent while simultaneously assimilating a new role relationship that is the inverse of the previous one. The person who had been depended upon in the recent or far past now has become the one who needs to be dependent.

Such a reversal may cause a great deal of stress in the children who are left to grieve for the loss of what had been and for what they expected would be in the future. What is lost in each relationship is a function of how far the children have advanced toward psychosocial maturity and the particular nature of the role relationship they have with the parent. An adolescent experiences a different pattern of losses when a parent dements than does a sixty-year-old on the verge of retirement, though both are subject to the same "canonical" pattern of losses that impede the resolution of grief as described above. Where the child is in his/her own life cycle will determine the nature of what is to be grieved and how daily life will change.

Young Children and Adolescents

Counselors will likely have to deal with a number of reactions on the part of young children and adolescents who may not be able to grieve the significant losses they experience when a relative has dementia. If it is a parent who has become impaired, young children may become frightened, confused, or regressed in reaction to the changed behavior they witness. The child may become hostile, uncooperative, do poorly in school, avoid the presence of the parent and keep friends away. Psychosocial development of the child is effected because normal role relationships change, and the processes whereby identification and self-esteem develop are potentially adversely effected by the loss of typical parent-child developmental opportunities. In addition, the ability of the care-giving parent to compensate to the child for the loss of the other, impaired parent is impeded as he/she must give care to the dementing parent. The attention that normally goes to a child has to be shared with a parent in need of assistance. Thus there is a potential reduction of this important component by which his/her attempts at competence, individualization, and growth are guided and rewarded. The child thus loses attention from both parents. The impact of the loss of such attention and guidance have not yet been fully assessed and evaluated but it would appear from clinical experience that the loss of some of the "idyllic" experiences of normal childhood can lead to anger, frustration, sadness, guilt, and other emotions that may require children to get counseling in order to cope successfully.

Younger children may also experience a limbo similar to the spouse's experience, a limbo of having a dad or mom who is physically present but emotionally and psychologically fading away. They may experience this on many levels of their relationship with the parent. For example, the parent who once could be counted on to help with homework or to help plan an outing or cook a meal can no longer meet that need of the child. A parent who could reflect about the impact his/her behavior would have on the child and others in the family can no longer do this and begins to behave in some frightening ways. The once-trusted parent may become a person who might yell at the child for no reason, display his/her genitals in public or in view of the child, or may embarrass the child by behaving in a bizarre fashion when they are together outside the home. The person who is physically present is doing things that are incongruent with the person he/she appears to be, forcing the child to separate continually from the emotional and cognitive components of the internalized parent, which had formerly been constant reliable attributes of the concept "mom" or "dad." Children also become fearful of the death of the parent and fearful that they or the other parent might become impaired as well. The once-secure life they may have known is transformed into one in which people are suddenly vulnerable and don't really live forever. Fears and phobias may develop as a result, and the world may come to be seen as unpredictable and full of impermanence.

Adolescents have many of the same experiences as younger children when a parent becomes demented but may react to the separation and loss in somewhat different ways. The developmental work of an adolescent is largely concerned with identity formation and the overcoming of identity confusion.[37] The developmental trend is toward gradual restoration of the trust in one's body and its functions that has been shaken by pubertal changes, and an evolution from parents to peer group as the essential supports and value givers. An adolescent must be allowed to proceed along this course slowly so that the requisite experimentation with varying identities can take place in a socially acceptable way during the moratoria that delay the onset of adulthood.[38] Having a parent with Alzheimer's or other progressive dementia is quite likely to have an effect on the facility with which this developmental work may be accomplished.

As Erikson[39] points out, the changing body identity of the adolescent can be quite a jolt, when the once-dependable and mastered physical self changes with puberty. The adolescent witnesses a parallel phenomenon in the parent whose once-predictable body becomes decreasingly under his/her control and a worrisome source of anxiety for the parent and family members. The once-reliable model of what physical development would result in can contribute to the adolescent's feelings of uncertainty as the brain's inability to control the body is seen in the parent's behavior.

Trends toward trying on different identities may also be adversely effected as the adolescent is forcibly withdrawn from the "psychosocial moratorium"[40] of phase-appropriate development and thrust into a family environment where everyone's help is needed. Attempts at identity formation may become casualties of the family's need to have the adolescent provide supervision of the impaired parent or younger children, to supplement the family income, assist the care-giving parent by taking over chores, and other household duties. Time with the peer group may not be available because of these domestic demands, nor may the adolescent be able to participate in social, athletic, vocational, community, or other activities that provide opportunities for socialization and development or trying on a mosaic of pieces in the identity formation. Indeed, an adolescent may decide that what the family needs is for him/her to take over more of the roles played by the impaired parent while maintaining an active school and social life.[41] Family conflict can develop when adolescent children feel stuck between the pressure to relieve the burdens of the care-giving parent and wanting to be free of care-giving tasks, or over which child of two is doing more to help out.[42]

For the adolescent, then, with a parent with Alzheimer's disease, separation and loss involve developmentally appropriate adjusting to the separation from and loss of a previous self (prepubertal) and the development of an identity that incorporates all previous identities.[43] Such an adolescent must adjust to the extra burden of separating from and losing a parent from whom he/she sought distance but not disappearance. It can be particularly difficult for an adolescent to lose a parent at a point when that parent could be appreciated in the context of a new, more peer-oriented relationship. Adolescents may also experience embarrassment with the disinhibition of behavior, especially any sexual displays, brought on by the parent's dementia, and may avoid the parent or refuse to bring friends home. Given the social patterns of this stage, such a reaction may place the teenager in conflict with the care-giving parent. The adolescent may want to spend time with friends, yet wish to do so away from home. The care-giving parent may understand this need yet require assistance in caring for the impaired parent. This leaves the adolescent with a difficult choice of what to lose—the peer group or the good feelings derived from assisting with family obligations.

Adult and Middle-aged Children

The concept of developmental lines[44] here again provides a valuable framework with which to examine the effect of dementias on the adult and middle-aged children of the patient. Even if the adult child is not the primary care-giver, dementia will have a profound impact on his/her life and the lives of his/her spouse and children. The emotional impact of experiencing the gradual mental deterioration of a parent while being unable to do anything to stop it produces internal distress and may have a stressful effect on the adult child's relationships in his/her own family. Both individual and interpersonal aspects will be discussed since so much of what is achieved during adult development is comprised of complementary growth in both areas.

Relationships to Parents

(Thirties through Forties)

- Evolution of adult-adult friendships.
- Reaction to the aging process in parents.
- Facilitation of parent's role as a grandparent.
- Mourning, integration of parent's death.

(Fifties and Beyond)

- Acceptance of reversal of roles, ability, and willingness to care for the aging incapacitated parent.
- Intrapsychic relationship to parental memories' effect on development.

Once a separate identity has been established the young adult in his/her twenties–thirties is expected to establish financial and emotional independence from his/her parents.[45] Normal development is further facilitated if the child becomes able to recognize and accept the limitations of the parents, and proceed to establish adult-adult relationships with them from an autonomous, independent yet emotionally connected position. When a parent develops dementia, however, the balance established during the twenties–thirties and thirties–forties—i.e., friendship and the pursuit of complementary developmental goals with parents—becomes fragile as role reversals and coping with a parent's illness and death become matters of immediate psychological concern. The adult child is therefore forced to cope with the loss of the relationship that had been evolving in the direction of mutual satisfaction toward maturity, and grieve the relationship that will never be. In relationships in which mutual development could not proceed because one or both partners was stuck trying to resolve the work of an earlier developmental level, the child may be forced to become more involved with that parent than he/she cares to. Additionally, if either or both individuals have not been able to develop along congruent and complementary paths along the appropriate line(s) of development, stress on the relationship will arise from the urgent need or pressure to give care. The incongruity inherent in the reversal of roles in such situations is even more stressful when the relationship has not achieved the developmental precursors necessary for this interdependent interaction pattern to succeed. Pressure to adjust in an environment of need and crisis can lead individuals and relationships to a state of collapse.

The care of a demented parent by adult children is a considerably stressful duty. Counselors will have to pay special attention to the impact of care giving on the life of the child of a parent with dementia. Marital and family stress, reduced job performance, anxiety, depression, withdrawal of interest from the spouse, children, and community affairs are but some of the reactions known to occur. Counselors will have to help the adult child cope with feelings and conflict that arise when a parent becomes demented, and do so according to the specific life circumstances of the child and the locus of the stress vis-a-vis his/her progress along developmental lines.

Case Example

Mr. and Mrs. Hodges decided to seek counseling about where to place her eighty-year-old mother who was suffering from Alzheimer's disease. They had determined that their ability to care for her had been exceeded by the growing behavioral, memory, and other problems her dementia presented. An additional dilemma was posed by the likelihood that Mr. Hodges could apply for a transfer to a geographic area they considered desirable as a location for their retirement living. If he were transferred now, at age sixty, their moving expenses would be paid by his employer, and they would have two additional years to spend in the community in which they had chosen to spend their later years. Such a plan would enable them to become established in that community, and to have a social network, friendship group, community interests, recreation, etc., into which they could plunge full-time when retirement was available to Mr. Hodges at age sixty-two. While such a move had obvious advantages for the Hodgeses, they were unsure about what was best for Mrs. Hodges's mother, Mrs. Gilliam. The long-term care facility they liked best, and which offered the best therapeutic program for Mrs. Gilliam, was located in their current hometown, though Mrs. Gilliam had moved there only five years before and had few friends. The only long-term care facility in the community to which the Hodgeses were moving had a special dementia program that they felt was inferior to the first facility's. The Hodgeses were unsure as to whether seeing Mrs. Gilliam every four to six months after they moved would adversely effect her behavior and emotions.

Counseling with the Hodgeses was concerned with clarifying these issues in light of their developmental needs both at the present time and in the future, and promoting an honest realistic discussion about their feelings as to whether they were ready to separate from the mother and how she might respond, given her personality and cognitive dysfunction. They decided that: (1) she would probably adapt well wherever she went to reside if she went there while her remaining social skills were functional; (2) they were inclined to accept the transfer because of all it offered them; (3) Mrs. Gilliam's memory was such that an absence of one day was like an absence of one month, so that not seeing her daughter every week would probably not be as significant for her as it would be for the daughter; and (4) they would feel better if Mrs. Gilliam resided in an environment where she could do best i.e.: flourish for as long as possible.

When a Grandparent Has Dementia

Colarusso and Nemiroff[46] propose that one of the developmental tasks adults face is to become comfortable with grandparenthood. If that is true, then children must undergo a reciprocal developmental process where the successful outcome is to adjust to being a grandchild. While most persons would consider this task easy to accomplish, it should be noted that not all grandparents and grandchildren have idyllic relationships. We must therefore evaluate the impact of having a grandparent with dementia in the grandchild's life against a realistic backdrop of what three-generational family life is actually like if we are to truly understand the grandchild's experience.

The age of the grandchild, relationships with the grandparent, relationships between the parents and grandparents, proximity to and frequency of visits with the grandparent, and other factors should be considered when appraising the impact on the grandchild. Whether or not the impaired grandparent lives with the grandchild and his/her parents, visits frequently, or is far away and is seen rarely, and how the parents are affected by their parent's dementia can make a difference in the grandchild's reaction and the impact the disease has on his/her life.

Younger children and adolescents who must share their house with a demented grandparent may experience a range of feelings when the grandparent comes to stay. Many respond very positively and become the family members with the best, most understanding relationships with the grandparents. If they have to give up their room, sacrifice special opportunities (like a vacation) or regular activities they may experience a change from having a positive feeling about the grandparent to feeling a siblinglike rivalry. On the other hand they may adjust graciously. The youngster may also wonder why grandfather's behavior is so strange and whether he/she (the child) caused it. It is not uncommon that some of the typical normal behavior of a child or teenager will cause increased anxiety, agitation, explosive outbursts, or complaints that "Steve was a bad boy today" to the parent, and the grandparent might come to be resented.

Children are usually aware of everyone's feelings and have some strong ones of their own. They therefore need to be included in any counseling the family undertakes, so that they can be encouraged to express themselves about family life as they experience it. "Grandpa is not the same, I wish he'd go back to being like he used to be" is the way one youngster expressed himself and then wanted to know whether he could do something or behave differently to "make grandpa come back." Explanations about why Grandpa is behaving like he is can help the child gain some understanding of what is happening, but the child must be helped at the same time to express any feelings about losing the Grandpa he/she knew before he became ill. Young children's questions about death may provide an appropriate opportunity if to discuss this issue on a level particularly suited to their developmentally appropriate ability to understand. Guthrie's recent work,[47] presents some of these issues in a way very beneficial for children's understanding of why Grandpa behaves the way he does. Van Ornum and Mordock[48] offer excellent insights for the counselor who will have to help children or adolescents cope with death as part of the experience of sharing a home with a demented grandparent.

Family circumstances sometimes make it necessary for an older dementia patient to live with an adult grandchild.

Case Example

Eighty-six-year-old Mrs. Hines lived with one of her two grown granddaughters after her progressive dementia made it dangerous for her to live alone. Her daughter and she had become estranged many years before, though this daughter's two children remained very close to their grandmother and felt that their mother's personality was to blame for the rift. They elected to have Mrs. Hines live in the house with one of them, and agreed that they would share her care. This they did for seven years until placement became necessary due to Mrs. Hines's considerable cognitive and physical deterioration. The two sisters visited their grandmother faithfully, and were able to encourage their mother to visit once to try and make peace with her mother before she died.

Counseling with this family was unique because the close relationship between Mrs. Hines and her granddaughters made them feel as if they were losing a parent to dementia, rather than a grandparent. They grieved this loss as Mrs. Hines became more disabled, and expressed the feeling that she had been more of a mother to them than had their own mother. They were able to feel satisfied that they had done the best that they could for Mrs. Hines.

A current phenomenon in the long-term care field is the increasing number of professional care-givers who become responsible for the care of an elderly relative. Many of these are women in their forties and fifties who must care for an aging parent who lives with or near them. In some instances, an aging, confused grandparent becomes the responsibility of a grandchild who, because he/she is a health-care worker, is presumed by the family to be the best candidate for the job. Such situations can produce enormous stress on the grandchild.

Case Example

Mrs. Madison is a professional nurse whose grandmother lived in a nearby community with Mrs. Madison's grandfather. The grandmother began to exhibit signs of confusion, lost the ability to care for herself, and would wander out during the day and night completely undressed. Her husband did not cooperate with any available community-based care services available in their community, so it was decided that the patient required placement in a long-term care facility. Mrs. Madison worked in a special care unit for persons with dementia at a nearby health-care facility, but was reticent about recommending that her grandmother be placed there. "My personal feelings were definitely in the way," she said. "I know my grandmother would get great care in our unit, but I felt that I'd have to apologize to my fellow workers each time my grandmother did something that wasn't normal." Because Mrs. Madison's parents were moving across the country at the same time to begin their retirement, she was left with the responsibility for the decisions about her grandmother's care and placement. She was told by her mother, who had completely cut off involvement with the grandmother due to her feelings about some old family secrets, that since she was a nurse she could take care of the situation and handle what her mother now called "minor problems" (she had previously responded to these problems as "major catastrophes"). Mrs. Madison's siblings were fearful for their own futures when their grandmother became confused; they believed she had a kind of insanity that was genetically determined. Mrs. Madison became very concerned over what to do, since she began to fear that if her grandmother lived a long time, she might have to care for her parents and grandmother in the future. Mrs. Madison's grandmother entered a skilled-nursing facility where, as fate would have it, Mrs. Madison was then employed. "At first I wouldn't let any of the nurse's aides touch her. I'd do all her care. My grandmother, who had been a lovely, kind woman, now would curse at me, spit at me, and bite me every day when I took care of her." When she realized what she was doing—carrying the burden of her family that everyone had transferred to her because she was a nurse and so "could take care of it"—she began the process of letting go. She made sure that her grandmother's medication was properly administered, and performed other duties as would be appropriate for her job, but she stopped providing direct physical care. Over a two-month period she was able to complete the separation process with no residual guilt and could ultimately leave to take a better position. The rest of her family, she says, has not yet dealt with grandmother's illness except by denial or inquiring through an occasional phone call as to whether she is still alive. In an interesting postscript Mrs. Madison realized that her great-grandmother had been demented like her grandmother was, and is "planning for the likelihood that I'll get dementia too."

When an Adult Child Develops Dementia

A most rarely seen clinical picture is one in which an older parent must contend with the unique and especially tragic circumstances of caring for an adult child with Alzheimer's or other dementia. It is especially heartbreaking to outlive one's children, and the loss of a child has been characterized as something from which a parent never recovers.[49] The longevity of the current generations of elderly persons makes it more common that parents in their seventies to eighties can have forty-five to sixty-five-year-old children who are at increasing risk for dementia.

Such a family situation presents particularly difficult dilemmas regarding care options, grief work, and the addition of the parent as a victim and casualty of the dementing disease.

Case Example

Ms. Harris is a fifty-two-year-old single female who has enjoyed a thirty-year career as a legal secretary. When her memory began to fail, she sought medical attention and was diagnosed as having Alzheimer's disease. It was concluded that she was unable to live alone for fear that she would injure herself or cause problems for her neighbors if she forgot to turn off her iron or stove. Having no other close relatives, she had no choice but to ask her eighty-seven-year-old mother whether they could live together. Her mother was a caring devoted woman, who had taken pride in her daughter's independence and success. She agreed to the arrangement in spite of her own significant medical problems. Though she had a history of cardiac disease, arthritis, and a mild hearing impairment, she continued to care steadfastly for her daughter for a number of years as the dementia progressed. Attempts to persuade her to get help, or consider placement in a long-term care facility, were politely but firmly refused. The mother's health continued to deteriorate as the physical and emotional stress of caring for her daughter became increasingly intense.

Counseling Considerations

Counseling families and family members can be undertaken with numerous orientations and procedures. Since most counselors preparing to provide counseling for family members of dementia patients are likely to be comfortable with particular theoretical and pragmatic positions about how to do family intervention, this discussion will not advocate for one or another of these established techniques. In this context, then, it is advantageous to examine some straightforward strategies by which to appraise the structure of the family as a system that may be able to provide care, and as a major variable in determining the emotional reaction of each member. Similarly, strategies for family intervention will be discussed.

Assessment

Whether a counselor is assisting an individual family member, a marital pair, siblings, or two generations of a family, it is helpful to obtain some information about the current status of the family system as well as some family history in order to shed light on the development of the family as an interpersonal system of relationships. A brief history can be obtained from a client by inquiring about the development of the spousal relationship or evolution of the family, and by noting the important milestones in the family's development (i.e., birth of children, death of the parents of each spouse, marital status of and closeness of adult children, grandchildren, retirement plans, etc.). It is especially important to place into historical perspective the onset of the behavioral changes brought on by dementia. The actual and potential support system should also be discussed. When counseling children, grandchildren, nephews, nieces, and other family members, it is also helpful to get some family history in order to put the patient and client in a family context and thereby avoid the tendency to see them as isolated individuals unaffected by the behavior of other significant persons in their lives.

Counselors might also find it helpful to inquire of care-giving relatives about how they became the care-giver. Were they like Mrs. Madison, "chosen" by the family, did they volunteer, were they seeking to renegotiate a relationship with the patient by assuming their care and demonstrating filial or sibling devotion or to create a debt of gratitude? Are they seeking "martyrdom" by assuming the care giving, or are they a "pseudocaretaker" who assumes an executive position and delegates responsibility to others?[50] Some may be spouses or only children of a widowed parent or may be in other ways the only alternative. Exploring the dynamics and realities by which a care-giver has been chosen frequently elicits many feelings the client has not had a prior chance to express. It is important to allow such ventilation if a realistic appraisal of future care-giving possibilities is to be determined, as when some of these feelings can be expressed, looked at, and understood, the client can opt for a different (perhaps less-stressful) emotional contract between him/herself and the patient.

Through the history and background gathered in the early part of counseling it is possible to get a feeling of each family member's perspective on things. Each relative may have a different viewpoint on a number of issues, and the nature of these disagreements as well as the points of concurrence should become known to the counselor.

Case Example

Mr. George Murchison and his brother James, along with their wives, consulted a counselor so as to be better able to cope with visits to their mother, an Alzheimer's-disease patient who resided in a skilled-nursing facility in a neighboring state. The brothers were part of a large family of siblings who seemed to be divided into two camps. One thought that their mother was well-cared-for and doing fine, but the clients were disturbed by the mother's acute, profound confusion when they visited her. Living outside the community where their mother and the rest of the family lived meant they could see her less frequently than their siblings. They were dubbed the "out of staters" to denote their peripheral status and were told that they had to visit every sixth week—no more and no less. A brief discussion of their family history and the history of their mother's dementia indicated that their youngest sibling, Mary, was very close (attached) to the mother. Because of her guilt over not being able to care for her at home she was overly involved at the nursing home to the point where she would listen to no criticism or questions about the patient's care. Mrs. James Murchison said that she was only one of the four clients who spoke to Mary because the other three worked all day. When Mary called each day to share the latest (and usually bad) news about the mother Mrs. Murchison was then supposed to communicate to her husband, brother-in-law, and sister-in-law. She said, "I guess I have to admit that I don't like doing this. I'd prefer not to be the messenger, but she won't even call and speak to her brothers. What's worse is that I was never accepted by their family except by George and his wife, and I guess I resent having to use what little time we have to speak with each other to be the intermediary of Mary's messages. We always end up feeling tense and unhappy when we talk about what Mary told me each day." This background information was useful for the counselor. He was able to inquire of the clients about their realistic expectations for change, given the control Mary had over things at the nursing home. The reality was that they felt ill at ease visiting as much as they did because they didn't know what to say or do with their mother when they visited. "We were such a big family," said James, "that neither I nor my brother spent much time with our mother. She was caring for the next younger kids that came along, so the sooner you were independent the better. Now, I don't even know what to talk to her about and she can hardly speak to me so I can understand her."

The next issue raised by the counselor in this initial interview was the selection of the problems they wished to solve. Counseling should be primarily oriented towards solving the difficulties that have arisen because a relative has become demented, and not towards attempting in-depth psychotherapy.[51] At times a counselor will be able to help clients with issues highlighted by the impact of dementia on the family, issues that reflect an underlying dysfunction in the family. In this case, Mrs. Murchison's role as the resentful messenger was chosen by this family as one issue they wished to solve. They also wanted to find a way to approach the nursing home about the behavior they saw in their mother that made their visits so frustrating, and wanted to get help deciding whether or not it was reasonable to insist that they visit when they could and not according to a schedule handed to them by another sibling.

With the Murchison family a historical problem had found new expression in the current difficulties caused by the patient's dementia, her need for care and visitation, and the impact of this reality on the already-existing relationships between the patient and her children as well as among the various siblings and their spouses. The counselor might therefore seek to discover during the assessment-oriented portion of early counseling sessions whether the emotional stresses reported by the family or discerned by his/her perceptive listening are new, continuing, or reactivated.[52] Knowledge of the nature of the stress experienced by the family can be of use in choosing appropriate goals with the client, and can help the counselor focus on the problem arising from the dementia when it is clearly evident—e.g., "How can we find out why Mother's behavior is so deteriorated when we visit?" Newer stresses can be presumed to be more amenable to problem-oriented intervention, and would be likely subjects for initial counseling sessions that sought to bring some early emotional relief.

Cohen[53] has presented a useful assessment protocol by which a counselor can appraise a family's capacity to develop plans to cope with the stressful effects of dementia. Not all families have the time, energy, finances, and other resources available to accomplish all the care giving they would like to do (or do what they think is expected of them by other relatives, neighbors, friends, etc.). Therefore, it can be very helpful to develop a realistic picture that serves as a guideline to help guard against unreasonable or impossible commitments by well-intentioned family care-givers who lack sufficient individual or community resources. Cohen suggests we assess:

The Impact on the Family | 63

1. The degree of organization (or disorganization) of the family system (or interpersonal support system).
2. Each family member's current understanding of and ability to understand medical and psychological problems.
3. The level of "dysfunction" and residual adaptive capacities of the patient.
4. The interpersonal disruption in the family caused by the patient's problem.
5. The degree of cooperation within the family.
6. The psychodynamics of the patient and each family member.
7. The presence of psychopathology that would preclude the cooperation of any of the family members (e.g., alcoholism, depression, thought disorders, impulse disorders, etc.).
8. The existence of major physical illness of a chronic or recurring type in any of the family members.
9. The current status of the marriage and dynamics of the marital relationship (whether the patient is a spouse of the client or the client is a care-giver relative and is married).
10. The nature of the family communication systems, the ways emotion are expressed, the role designations and behavior, the family myths, the family secrets, the family image of itself.
11. Traumatic events that have affected the family in the recent or remote past.
12. Recent or recurrent crises in the life of any family member.

Each family will have its own pattern of stressful and helpful components on each of these dimensions; these will yield an overall impression for the counselor about how ready a family is to undertake care, and how much care can realistically be undertaken. Once the family's capacity to provide care has been evaluated, their own plans can be discussed with regard to: (1) what they can realistically expect to do; (2) what they will need to obtain from community-based service providers; (3) how they feel about accepting help; (4) how they feel if too large a gap between need and resource availability exists for the patient to remain at home; and (5) how they will handle any family conflict over the way to provide the best-available care appropriate to the patient's level of need (e.g., to institutionalize or not).

Intervention

Zarit[54] suggests a modified version of the nine-step counseling model discussed earlier as a useful method of reducing care-giver burdens in family care-givers to a dementia patient. It is especially useful to help with care-giving stresses, and in reducing the disruptive effect the behavior of the dementing person is having on the care-giver. The problem-solving strategy he advocates utilizes objective, behavioral terms to *identify problem behaviors* (how often and when does the problem behavior occur), *generate solutions* through brainstorming, *selecting a solution* and airing pros and cons about it from among the possibilities discussed, *cognitive rehearsal* of the solution to identify blocks that might prevent its working, *encouragement* to carry out the plan, and *evaluation* of the outcome. Successful plans are carried out, and unsuccessful ones are modified until they are effective. This approach can also be used to help families solve particular problems about care giving, planning, and execution of care plans, exploring options, etc., in addition to intervention with discreet behavioral events. It is an approach designed to mobilize and expand the care-giver's problem-solving skills. The nine-step counseling model described in chapter 4 is a slightly more expanded but congruent method to help care-givers identify a problem area, narrow down their possible responses, explore feelings about each one, and choose an option that feels right.

Grieving

As a result of many emotional difficulties that can be a result of the separation process described earlier in this chapter, a counselor may have to assist the family member(s) in understanding and working through the peculiar grief reaction families report when experiencing the disease. The spouse of a dementia patient said, "When Al died, I had no more need to grieve. I was relieved, liberated from my suffering as he was from his. But while he was alive, I grieved everyday." Grief without crippling guilt while the patient is alive is the often-elusive goal toward which counseling the family should aspire. Helping family members separate is a slow process during which many feelings emerge. These feelings are often strong, but frequently defy articulation. Marion Roach[55] provides some definition of what family members, spouses, children of various ages, and grandchildren, might be feeling. She described the disease (Alzheimer's) as "careering through the family, leaving them ... standing speechless and stunned by rage. We look at one another, we look at the victim, and we look away for help. The ability to panic leaves the victim; it swarms over the family.... I hate this disease."

Counseling can be a very beneficial intervention to help family members cope with feelings like Marion Roach's or Myrna Doernberg's achingly clear emotional turmoil. Family members' particularly unique grieving process requires much support and assistance while they endure the separation, anger, sadness, guilt, blame, and mourning that cascade over them as they watch their beloved person disappear. It is a uniquely private grief that requires a nonjudgmental, supportive, accepting, witness who understands what people do not acknowledge—that dementia renders the patient "familiar and profoundly changed, at once there and absent."[56] It is the difficult and often-delicate task of the counselor to help the grieving relative let go of what is absent while holding on to what is there, all the while not letting go of or clutching tightly at too much. Letting go too soon makes the patient feel abandoned; the family member feels guilty and resentful that the patient is still alive. If what is gone is not let go of, the patient is pressured to be the person he/she no longer is and thus disappoints and fails; the family member feels intense guilt for not doing enough and angry that the patient isn't responding.

Another painful private grief is experienced by those who share feelings of love and friendship with the patient but who have no legal or otherwise societally sanctioned relationship with him/her. Lifelong companions or persons who have developed spousal interconnections in later life without marriage, or even cohabitation, experience the same grieving for their vanishing companion, but receive less social support than spouses do because they occupy no traditional role. Counselors may have a difficult time recognizing the depth of their relationship to the patient if biases against heterosexual or homosexual relationships among the aged cloud their vision and prevent them from recognizing the pain of the grieving partner. This partner's grief is no less intense, and his/her loss is no less grievous. These are family relationships in the truest interpersonal sense, whether the partners have shared a platonic or sexual relationship. A counselor's biases about aging and sexuality, or vulnerability to stereotypes about how "proper older persons" ought to behave, cannot be allowed to deprive the grieving patient and partner from receiving a full complement of help.

Adult children of dementia patients may require counseling help to cope with the many conflicting feelings they might have about the deterioration and death of their parent. In some instances, adult children who assume some responsibility for coordinating and/or providing care for the patient must try to resolve feelings about lose-lose situations brought on by conflicts over medical care decisions for demented parents that could prolong life—and dementia—for a longer period of time.

Adult children of dementia patients may require active assistance in coping with their grief. Counselors can help identify where in the grief process the client is found and explain the canonical nature of the grief felt by the families of dementia victims. Counselors can let them express their ambivalent feelings and help them accept these confusing emotions, as many persons cannot understand how they can feel one way and yet another with equal intensity. They may have to be reassured that this is not a sign of being crazy or even that such feelings are not an indication that they have dementia (a common response in some family members when they feel unfamiliar and disturbing feelings). Adult children may also require support in coming to terms with their impending orphanhood and the fact that they will move up one step toward the front line of mortality—perhaps to the very front—when the parent dies. Thus, as an adult child grieves the loss of and separation from the parent who is fading away, he/she must also contemplate his/her own aging and mortality. Clients may find this confusing, feel disturbed that they are thinking about themselves at a time when their parent is in such distress, or recognize understandable feelings of resentment about this particular impact of their parent's dementia. Since people tend to be less tolerant of others if they are intolerant of themselves, counseling can provide relief to the adult child by helping him/her accept these feelings and reduce internal, unsatisfactory judgment against the self. This in turn can produce more acceptance and tolerance of the demented parent's behavior and disabilities.

Adult children may have difficulties talking about their family. They might even express the thought that to talk about the family to an outsider *feels* wrong in spite of their objectively felt need for help. This may become an issue especially when counseling shifts away from concrete service finding issues to an examination of feelings. As children grow up and internalize the socially and morally imposed obligations of family life, they also acquire some unconscious and subtly imposed ones. These latter rules are rarely articulated but are learned through repeated exposure to subtle cues. One such obligation of family life is the need to keep "family secrets," a contract which may be violated when invisible loyalties are taken outside the family to be viewed by strangers when help is needed.[57] (In a recent phenomenon, loyalty can also be imposed from outside the family, such as when governmental agencies, hospitals, long-term care facilities, and other societal institutions demand that adult children become the care system of first resort and presume that they will take on the burden of care for aged, infirm parents no matter what the relationship has been over the years.) When in counseling, adult children may wish to present only the public face that they have been taught to portray many years before, and not expose critical, angry, or other dissatisfied feelings about a parent, sibling, or other relative. The client who feels this way will require reassurance that the invisible loyalties that constrain them are part of a contract they did not knowingly sign, and that having angry feelings about a relative does not mean one doesn't love him/her. The counselor can also suggest that the client might discover that those "secrets" he/she was supposed to keep from outsiders might not be as damning or onerous as family mythology might have had it.

An adult child may also feel, or be given the message that he/she is bad or ungrateful if unable to reciprocate to the demented parent in an identical way for the care given to him/her as a child. This "ledger balancing"[58] is an unrealistic expectation, as it is impossible for the parent to be repaid in concrete terms, whether or not he/she becomes demented. When the child has been the object of affection, caring, and protection, these may have been rendered and accepted with a hidden, implied "agreement" which stipulated that the devotion shown to the young child would be repaid in kind when the parent became dependent.[59] But earlier periods of family life cannot be re-created, and parental and child roles cannot be reversed. Counselors may have to help adult children understand that a direct payback to a parent for all he/she did is not possible and that in spite of actual feelings of gratitude or guilt, the child can repay only in spirit, but not in kind, with fairness and justice. But he/she will be endlessly frustrated, and so will future generations, if he/she attempts to undo the essential asymmetry of the parent-child relationship[60] because an intergenerational legacy of unpayable debts will be perpetuated.

Counseling children

Children may need more assistance in finding a forum in which to express their feelings than they will in perceiving what is going on in their family. The sensitivity, insight, and notoriously refreshing honesty children possess make them helpful participants in family counseling. Their participation further ensures that the patient's illness (whether parent, grandparent, etc.) will not be treated as a mysterious, taboo subject within the context of family life. Children can be wonderfully understanding, tolerant, accepting, and even exemplary in the way they cope with the impact of having a demented relative in their lives. This is especially so if adults around them act likewise. A child's perceptions may depend on his/her cognitive capacities and mental organization at the time, and better understanding can be gained from open discussions about their reasoning as to why Grandma behaves a certain way. Family counseling creates a regular opportunity for the child to share his/her outlook on the events happening in the family's life, and to experience positive conflict resolution, alliance formation, and other family-strengthening processes along with the rest of the family. The child might also utilize counseling to learn how he/she can help with the family's care responsibilities. It is common that small children relate very well to cognitively impaired adults perhaps because they are not as aware of disabilities as adults are and can form relationships based on congruent and complementary emotional and cognitive functioning. One family reported that their ten-year-old daughter was the only person from whom the cognitively impaired grandmother would take directions about bathing. Whereas she would physically resist her son or daughter-in-law's attempts to get her to take a bath, the ten-year-old would simply say, "Come on, Grandma, it's time to take a bath" and Grandma would smile and comply.

Children may feel sad about the condition of their relative but not about the same aspects as adults do. They may find it difficult to understand why adults are sad about what "Grandma can't do" or "what Grandma has lost," since they can relate quite well to their relative in spite of the cognitive impairment. They might even understand his/her behavior better than the adult can. A child might be sad that Grandpa can't remember when dinner time is, or that he says he's lost, and may also feel his/her parent's sadness about Grandpa's condition. Children can be helped by counselors to talk about what makes them feel sad, angry, etc.

Adolescents and older children may find counseling a useful experience in spite of some initial misgivings (some based on the invisible loyalties discussed earlier or because of fears that someone might be reading their minds). Family or individual counseling can help the youngster express feelings of frustration about how life has changed since the relative became impaired, and to express fears, feelings of sadness, and/or anger about losing their father, grandmother, etc. Counselors can encourage children to ask questions about the disease and what the future holds, and help resolve family conflicts to reduce fighting. Adolescents may be particularly receptive to some time alone with the counselor at the end of a family counseling session (or at another time) to share feelings about their parents in a safe atmosphere. The counselor may wish to encourage the adolescent to express his/her feelings with the parents at a later date, and may help by using cognitive rehearsal, role-playing, etc. They may also wish to talk about grieving in private at first, so that they become familiar with their feelings and reduce the risk of embarrassment should they cry in front of the entire family. It is not unusual for an adolescent or young adult to have within him/herself many strong, complex feelings about a parent or grandparent that nobody else in the family is able to get in touch with or express.

3

Communicating with the Demented Elderly Person

A major source of frustration in taking care of a demented person is caused by the wide array of communication difficulties that are primary disabilities in dementing disorders. Patients and care-givers give evidence that they feel the normal flow of information they have come to expect from within themselves, or from other people with whom they are communicating, has been somehow changed.

As usual and habitual ways of exchanging information with another person cease to be effective, previously effortless communication activities become difficult and tedious. Family members and professional caregivers will have to learn to understand the often confusing utterances or behavioral signals demented people use to express themselves, and to change the ways they speak so that the patient can understand the true meaning of what they are communicating.

General Hints about Communication with Demented Persons

1. Never assume that they don't know what you are talking about when you speak in their presence. A demented person retains the capacity to understand language well after he/she cannot speak intelligibly, and can understand the emotional content of facial and other cues (anger, sadness, etc.)[1]

2. As you would not speak about any patient to another individual while that patient is present, so also should you avoid talking about a demented individual to another while the patient is present.

3. Do not hold conversations with another person in close proximity to a demented person as if he/she weren't there. The patient's difficulties in understanding what is being said may make him/her think that he/she is the subject of the conversation. This can lead to

angry reactions by the patient if, for example, you are talking to a coworker about someone at whom you are angry and the patient believes you are referring to him or her. Such a misperception can lead to aggression by the patient or other emotional reactions.

4. Use short, simple sentences or questions.

5. Avoid the use of pronouns (*him, her*) and use proper names that the patient can recognize or is familiar with.

6. Talk about observable, actual occurrences rather than abstract, philosophical issues that may be difficult to understand or communicate about. This can lead to feelings of being "stupid" or "less than I used to be" in the patient.

7. Position yourself at eye level with the patient, preferably seated, so that the patient does not feel that you might terminate the conversation quickly. This fear increases pressure to "perform," in this case to be verbally fluent, and can therefore heighten the patient's anxiety and diminish functional memory ability.

8. Allow the patient time to listen, comprehend, think, formulate, and express a response to what you have said. Be careful not to communicate impatience or annoyance if communication takes longer. It probably will. If you manifest impatience, the patient may feel that you are angry or disappointed. In the former case he/she may respond with angry feelings; in the latter, he/she may choose not to risk the loss of self-esteem that comes with disappointing people whom you respect, and the patient may stop communication should this occur.

9. Reduce background noise and other stimuli that compete for the demented patient's attention and make it difficult to pay attention to your message. In middle-stage patients, things like noisy jewelry, telephones ringing, public-address systems, and busy nurses' stations or hallways can further impede the patient's already-compromised communication ability.

10. Be direct in your messages. Do not expect the patient to draw inferences from what you say. For example, if you are too busy to speak with the patient but will talk to him/her in an hour say, "I can't talk now, but I will see you at twelve-thirty" rather than "Does it look like I have time now? See me later when I'm free."

11. Avoid metaphor and analogy. Dementia patients are unable to abstract the properties of two things and establish their similarity or mutual class membership (e.g., that apples and bananas are "fruit").

12. Dementia patients think literally. Saying "Why don't you jump into the shower" may provoke a response such as "I'm afraid to, I might fall." Use descriptive terms that are unambiguous. ("Put on your green blouse" rather than "get dressed now.")

13. Restate and paraphrase your message if it isn't understood.[2] This will allow you to formulate your communication in such a way as to be understood by each particular patient as best he/she can, given the progression of his/her dementia.

14. Speak in a low-pitched, audible tone of voice with appropriate animation, intonational cues, and gestures. Verbal communication relies on all of these cues, and it is helpful for the patient to receive a stream of communication that contains as many of the normal channels of meaning as possible.[3] In this manner the patient can utilize a number of different cues to decode the message if the meanings of individual words are forgotten.

15. Remember and utilize the nonverbal elements of communication to enhance the patient's readiness to listen to or understand your message. Touch, facial expression, posture, head movements, eye contact, gesture, and position relative to the patient help communicate emotional messages about how the interlocutor is regarded and what feelings are to be conveyed. Be careful to touch demented patients only after trust has been established, and do so slowly, gently, and in full sight of the patient.

16. Assess the patient's ability to hear by watching whether your speech is audible. Many older persons suffer an age-related hearing loss that makes hearing others a difficult thing. We sometimes forget that dementia patients can have age-related physical difficulties as well as cognitive dysfunction. Be aware of visual deficits as well, and be prepared to compensate for these by changing lighting, relying less on visual cues, removing sources of glare, and making sure you can be seen.

17. Avoid becoming overexcited, using wild gestures, or being overly demonstrative as this can cause the patient to become alarmed and anxious. Dementia patients "absorb" care-givers' moods easily.

18. Provide cues and help the patient find the "lost" word while they are talking. When a patient describes a concept instead of using a noun, give them the word. For example if the patient says, "I'm looking for my, you know it's on my arm and I look at it" you can say, "Your watch?"

19. Dementia patients can read words even after they have lost some of the meanings of a word or phrase. Ambiguous sentences can cause real problems. A sign saying "EXIT" can be interpreted to be conveying a command, rather than just labeling a means of egress.

20. Attend to the words and the emotional message you are getting. If the person sounds upset while he/she is talking, or begins to cry, respond to the emotion you are seeing.

21. Ask one question or give one direction at a time. Use short sentences (five to ten words in sequence) rather than long paragraph-length utterances.

22. If the patient loses the thread of a story, or is unable to complete a sentence (e.g., pauses, looks at you, goes on to another topic), repeat the last phrase he/she said to prompt memory. If the patient cannot retrieve the sentence, paraphrase what he/she was saying and help him/her continue. If these are unsuccessful, do not pressure the patient for too long. He/She will probably have forgotten the idea by then.

23. Ask "yes" or "no" questions when appropriate, (e.g., "Does it hurt?" "Do you like the music?") but do not confine all your utterances to this category. Allow the patients to use remaining communication abilities in the framework of conversations with you. ("How do you like this dessert?")

24. The development of language comprehension precedes production in human development; it also remains longer when dementia occurs. Therefore, assume that the patient understands more than he/she can say, especially with regard to emotional messages.[4]

25. Observe the patient for signs of restlessness or withdrawal such as agitation (foot movements and handwringing), restless eye movements or continuous scanning of the room, becoming loud or argumentative, and frowning.[5]

26. Help the patient become tolerant of his/her communication difficulties. Support remaining skills and encourage their use. Reassure the patient that you'll take the time to listen.

27. Observe dementia patients to see how they communicate with each other and with care-givers. Get an idea of their vocabulary, sentence structure, and normal communication patterns so that you have a context by which to understand them better. Remember they are using a language, i.e., rule-governed communication. It is our job to understand and learn the rules of their communication so we

can become more adept at helping the patients use all their remaining communication ability as a means of personal expression and social adaptation.

I would like to close this discussion by relating a most remarkable instance of communication. It illustrates how we linguistically adept and cognitively unimpaired people can miss the significance of communication available to those who will persist with communication in spite of their dementia.

I was walking down the corridor of a long-term care facility when I spotted two older men, presumably residents of the nursing home, engaged in what appeared to be an animanted discussion. My vantage point did not allow me to see their faces, or hear their words, but I could see their gestures, body language (head movements, relationship of their heads as they walked), and other behavior. It looked as if they were engaged in a heated discussion of some kind, and reminded me of what I would see as a boy when I lagged behind my father and his colleagues who were inevitably discussing some gravely important issue or world event. The two gentlemen paused in their tracks and one leaned against the wall while the other faced him as they continued to converse. I approached them and could hear their voices but could not make out what they were saying. I strained my hearing so that I might discreetly eavesdrop on their conversation, my curiosity rationalized as a desire to do some "scientific observation" of what two apparently healthy men in a nursing home talk about. I fully expected to overhear a hallway bull session about the food, television, another resident, one or both of their families, or even the score of the last night's baseball game.

What I in fact did hear and see was two men engaged in the mutual exchange of phonation-sounds that were the closest thing to a string of nonsense syllables strung together I had ever heard uttered by human beings. This was not the "word salad" of schizophrenics or the sentences of demented people that start out somewhere and end up either nowhere or on a different subject than that of the opening phrase of the utterance. These men were simply exchanging sounds. But they did so with all of the appropriate facial expressions, gesture, and body language of a "normal conversation," and that apparently was sufficient to allow these two to feel that they were communicating. Their faces showed signs of what I took to be pleasure and interest, they showed and used moderate voice tone, and each looked at the person speaking to him, waited for him to finish, and then picked up his end of the conversation.

I checked with staff to see whether either spoke a language unfamiliar to me and was told that both of these demented men were native-born English speakers who had lived in the same rural part of New York State where the facility was located. Had it not been for the lack of identifiable English words, their communication behavior would otherwise have been indistinguishable from what one could see on any main street in the towns near where they lived.

As I drew near enough to be a factor in their environment, one looked up at me, smiled graciously, and gave me a sheepish look as if to say to me: "Look, it may not be profound, but we understand each other just fine." It *was* a profound lesson about how people with dementia are able to adapt to communication impairments and engage in interactions we as nonimpaired care-givers would readily and perhaps erroneously misjudge as nonsensical and meaningless.

4

Counseling Older Persons

This chapter is included to give an orientation and a context for counseling intervention around Alzheimer's disease and similar disorders. Since the incidence of Alzheimer's and related disorders increase with age, it is probable that persons doing counseling with victims of these conditions will be working with many people over age sixty.

The Basic Nine-Step Counseling Model[1]

1. Understanding the Client

During this initial step, the counselor gets to know and tries to understand the client. This is done by taking into account the individual's history, family dynamics, cultural and ethnic factors, cohort realities (age and historical epoch during which client has grown up and developed), source(s) and degree of stress and stress-reduction resources available at present for each domain in the life space (e.g., physical changes of aging, income level, social supports, cognitive and emotional status). At this beginning point of the counseling process it is necessary to remember that:

A. The client existed before coming to see a counselor and has that personal history as an internal point of reference from which to begin counseling. The counselor should be aware of that reference point.
B. Each person has *strengths* and positive attributes that typically bring about success, and *problem areas,* in which he/she expresses lack of success or frustration of effort. While the counselor may be "problem oriented" or looking for what is "broken" so it can be fixed, the client may wish to demonstrate first that he/she is a competent person and not in need of re-

pair. When this is recognized by the counselor, the client will be more likely to open up about the difficulties that necessitated intervention.

C. One must remember that among the current generations of elderly there are many clients who will be adamant about not wanting "free" help because it reminds them of being on "relief" as many were during the Great Depression, for many a sign of personal shame and failure. While younger counselors and other professionals recognize the many gains in the area of programs for older persons and the greater variety of social and medical services available to those with limited means, the worldview of the client must be understood and respected, and treated with dignity.

2. Establishing Rapport

The counselor must appraise the client's comfort level about talking with a stranger about problems and feelings. There will be a great deal of individual variation among clients. Some elderly are very pleased with such help (i.e., have greater dependency needs that they recognize and do not find uncomfortable), while others resist help. Rapport helps to get the process moving and establishes the presence of trust and mutual understanding. Three components are required for rapport to be established. These are:

A. Empathy:
Understanding the deepest feelings, frame of reference, and worldview of the client. The counselor maintains separation but "feels with" the client.
B. Respect:
A true belief that the client has worth as a person as he/she presently is. This is not equivalent to liking everything the client says or being in agreement with it. This can have enormous therapeutic impact. As Comfort has observed, "The traditional and intuitive social integrator for the problems of loss in age is respect."[2]
C. Concern:
Taking the client and the problem(s) he/she presents seriously. This is shown by being mentally and physically attentive.

3. Defining the Problem

It is usually helpful to ask the client to state the problem to be discussed as he/she sees it. This allows the client to set the agenda in a way that reflects his/her ease and comfort with topics for counseling.

Dialogue:

Mrs. Bloom was a seventy-six-year-old woman who had recently become forgetful. She came to a geriatric psychologist because as she put it, "I'm embarrassed by forgetting things. Why, I even forgot the number of your office while I was coming over here!"

COUNSELOR: Do you feel embarrassed to tell me about that difficulty?

MRS. BLOOM: Yes. I had a wonderful memory. I worked for the State Social Service Office and I remembered every name that was in my files. I could say hello to all of them by name. This problem with my memory is terrible, I feel so ashamed. Why can't I remember better?

COUNSELOR: What can we do together to help you feel less embarrassed?

MRS. BLOOM: Well, I don't think this is really due to anything serious, probably just my age, you know, but I'd like to know how to help myself feel better by remembering better.

Notice that Mrs. Bloom defined the problem as one concerning how she felt about herself (shame) rather than as a memory problem per se. Therefore, the focus of the first counseling session was on her self-esteem, her need to get help while maintaining some working defenses, e.g., denial, rationalization ("It's my age"), and gathering some information as a first step in discovering a possible etiology for the memory disorder. At the end of the first session Mrs. Bloom agreed that some laboratory studies (blood and urine) would be a good way to begin to explore the cause(s) of her problem. Because of her focus on her self-esteem, a full-fledged evaluation to rule out Alzheimer's disease was not felt to be appropriate until it could be suggested in the context of a later conversation after the client felt more comfortable and had dealt further with her embarrassment.

Mrs. Bloom illustrates very well the admonition counselors often hear that advises, "Meet clients where they are." This means that for counseling to have a high probability of success at the outset, the client should be allowed to choose what issue or stressor in his/her life shall be the first one addressed in the counseling interaction. This choice is likely to reflect the client's perception of what is an appropriate or pressing but not excessively disturbing topic of concern. Although not necessarily the crucial or most pressing issue from the counselor's viewpoint, it is nevertheless the most comfortable point of departure for the client and as such represents a choice which deserves respect, affirmation, and cooperation.

4. Setting a Goal

Asking a question such as "What would you like to see happen as a result of what we do together?" or "Do you have an outcome in mind toward which we can work?" is an efficient and democratic way of goal setting. Older persons like Mrs. Bloom who have strong feelings of autonomy at the core of their self-esteem ought to be treated as coworkers in counseling, and not as beneficiaries of the counselor's "wisdom." People seem to evaluate their circumstances more positively if they have had a hand in choosing them. But most of all, people who are actively involved in goal setting are more likely to succeed and obtain gratification for their success if they will be able to get credit for the outcome. Giving any client an equal voice in choosing a goal for counseling promotes self-esteem, a sense of control over the environment and enlists the elder in a "team effort" where he/she is ego-involved in the outcome.

Elderly people who enjoy being dependent on others, and who feel that their efforts are typically ineffective will likely try to have the counselor set the goal unilaterally. "After all," they'll say, "you're the expert. That's why I came to you." Such seductions, while flattering to a counselor's ego, can set the stage for later difficulties since none of us are omnipotent or omniscient. We are bound to fail to live up to such expectations at some point. Moreover, encouraging that opinion sets the stage for continued feelings of helplessness and incompetency on the part of the client. If the counselor chooses the goal and it is achieved, the client loses because he/she chose the wrong person to trust. A success will reflect positively on the counselor but will not bring any credit to the client. These dynamics encourage more dependency and pessimism on the part of the client, which continues the cycle of helplessness, failure and continued dependency.

5. Clarifying Issues

This step relies on the counselor's ability to "hear" what the client is saying in even the most disguised, abstruse, or convoluted manner. The counselor must study the feelings of the client, noticing any contradictions between what is said and what is indicated by emotional communication (intonations, body language, gestures, tears, a raised voice), by refusal to discuss certain topics, and by the use of prohibitive, negative, or evaluative terms—*should, can't, must, never, always, good, bad*—for oftentimes a client will communicate more about how he/she feels through nonverbal cues than verbal ones. These should be carefully pointed out during counseling.

Counseling the elderly requires that five basic assumptions be understood with regard to attending to feelings. These are:

A. Feelings are neither good nor bad.
B. Everyone has a right to his/her own feelings.
C. Feelings always seem appropriate when seen in the context of the client's worldview.
D. Feelings are not dangerous, though actions can be.
E. Denying a feeling does not make it disappear or lose its ability to influence behavior.

It has been noted elsewhere[3] that a person's comfort with emotion is often a function of his/her "generational psyche," that is, how a society felt about emotional expression in each generation, and how these values were inculcated in children by parents, teachers, role models, and the culture (literature, etc.) of the time. Veterans of the 1960s era when people were encouraged to express their feelings ("let it all hang out") might find it difficult to relate to how thoroughly people reared in previous generations were taught that emotional expressions were immature, unmanly, selfish, self-indulgent, childish, and a reason to feel guilt. Counselors should therefore bear in mind that just as the feelings of the client should not be negated, denied, suppressed, minimized, judged, or evaluated, neither should the client be pressured, embarrassed, browbeaten, manipulated, or otherwise forced to express a feeling or admit to one. Many elderly clients do not agree that the cathartic release of emotion will bring relief; they are sure, to the contrary, that such expressions will begin as endless flow of painful, embarrassing feelings, or won't help ("What good will it do to cry about those bad memories?"). Clients must always be allowed to determine a level of emotional expression that is both comfortable and therapeutic for themselves. Counselors can guide, encourage, and reassure; it may be counterproductive and even harmful to push or drag a client into an emotional mine field. The client will venture out when he/she is ready. Speaking of the elderly, Alex Comfort has advised:

> There indeed are those who suppress emotion or their hurt, but there are also those whose self-esteem depends on being in control and who remain so out of self-respect rather than out of fear of losing that control. The old and the young may indeed need to be helped to express (feelings), but particularly in the old expressions need not be spectacular.... We should neither react critically to those whose control genuinely fails nor—and this is now a more common error among junior counselors—be disappointed if we cannot induce an emotional response beyond the calm statement of feelings.[4]

6. Listing Alternatives

"What are the ways by which you could achieve your goal?" By this straightforward question the client is focused on paths toward a successful outcome. It can be a help to the client and validating of his/her positive self-esteem to see whether or not the client has faced the same or a similar problem before in his/her life, and to inquire about how the problem was solved at that time. If possible, might a similar strategy or method be used now? This is another, more direct way of evaluating how stresses in the life space have been reduced in the past and whether these ways are still available. If they are, then the client will be able to evaluate whether social stereotypes about aging, for example, are preventing the use of lifelong resources.

Dialogue

MR. BROOKS: I must confess to you that I really don't like living in Miami. I don't have much in common with the people in our condominium development. My wife and I haven't found any couples who like literature and good movies, and we miss our friends back home in Michigan. It is getting us depressed, tense, and angry with each other, though we agree about this feeling I'm telling you about. I don't need the stress, it aggravates my heart condition.

COUNSELOR: If you feel that way, have you thought about moving, or even going back to Michigan?

MR. BROOKS: Oh yes, we sure have. But people think you're crazy if you aren't happy here. My children told us to move here after I retired. They said that we would love it, there'd be so many people like us that we'd make many new friends and forget the people back home. Well, I don't mind telling you that in my mind this is no paradise for old people. But if you say that, people treat you like a heretic. "How dare you not love it here"—like all old people are supposed to love it in Miami.

COUNSELOR: Do you feel that it's abnormal for an older person not to like it here, or is that what society wants you to believe? If you don't like it, can you move to where you'd be happier?

MR. BROOKS: You're the first person down here I've met who thinks that how I feel is OK.

COUNSELOR: Let's talk about your options. How do you feel about living elsewhere in Miami? Would you prefer going back to Michigan?

If old solutions are not available due to resource depletion in any domain, new alternatives must be thought of and listed. For example, if an older man with heart disease wishes to but can't care for his ailing wife, home health assistance might be considered, along with long-term care placement, living with a relative who could provide the care, etc. The viability of these choices will be a function of the actual pattern of care needed and at resources are reliably available to the couple.

7. Exploring Alternatives

The list of alternatives generated in step 6 is next evaluated according to the possible positive and negative outcomes. Thus, Mr. Brooks listed the good and bad consequences of each of his alternatives, and decided that the positive outcomes on his social life and friendships if he moved to Michigan were outweighed by an overriding negative one—his health could not tolerate living in the cold North.

Each alternative can be assessed for positive and negative outcome, and the possibilities discussed explored and reevaluated. In Mr. Brooks's case, considerations of the alternatives in this way helped him decide that it was not crazy to want to move, and that there were many positive factors associated with living in a warm climate where he could remain mobile and healthy. He needed only to change where he lived if life were to possess a higher quality of social experience for himself and his wife. With his thinking about the problem systematically reorganized and alternatives logically discussed, he could feel more relaxed, less angry, and move on to step 8.

8. Reaching a Conclusion

Evaluating the positive and negative aspects of each alternative helps the client list the alternatives in the order of their desirability. This usually means that options have been considered not as all-or-nothing, black-and-white choices, but rather as mixtures of positive and negative components. The choice of an alternative requires that the client deal with the way he/she will cope with the (inevitable) negative aspects of even the most desirable positive choice. Mr. Brooks's list had three alternatives, which were (in order), to stay in Miami but relocate to a community more congruent with his needs; stay where he was; or return to Michigan. He decided that he would try to see his friends in the summer by visiting his hometown, and invite them to visit him in the winter months. These compromises make the negative aspects of his choice more tolerable, though he didn't get everything he wanted. After suitable research he found a new place to live that had people with whom Mr. Brooks could share discussions about books, attend movies, and talk about things other than how their children neglected them and the location of their latest aches and pains. His stress was greatly reduced and he and his wife ceased their incessant arguments.

9. Providing Closure

Once a choice is elected, counseling is set to reach its final step: closure. This usually means terminating the counseling relationship, though with many elderly persons and their families there will be multiproblem situations requiring prolonged counseling. In these cases, once a problem has been solved, client and counselor can begin at step 3 ("Defining the Problem") and go through the intervening steps for each problem in turn until the need for counseling no longer exists.

Such a process may require referral to other resource people in the community if a given problem calls for expertise the counselor (or the agency) does not possess. Referrals to another provider can be made as part of steps 6 and 7, or as part of the process of closure with the client. In the latter case feedback by the client and/or subsequent resource person help to provide closure for the counselor and client alike. Clients can also be requested to make periodic follow-up phone calls or visits to update the counselor until contact is totally stopped by mutual choice. An invitation to call upon the counselor again if help is needed says, "the door is always open for you here." This is an important message to many elderly persons who come to enjoy contacts with helpers of various kinds, and for whom visits to professionals may constitute the bulk of their social contacts. With this message the client is told that solving a problem does not necessarily mean a permanent end to the relationship that has evolved.

Except in cases where a decision presents a clear danger to the client, his or her family, neighbors, etc., "the client is the one who makes the final decision because it is his problem, his choice and his life.... The counselor should respect the choice even if it is unwise [because] the choice is always wise in the context of the client's worldview.[5] If the client decides not to make a choice, this choice must also be respected.

Following are some examples of counseling intervention in which these principles are applied:

Case Example

Mr. Meyer, an eighty-six-year-old writer with mild dementia was a regular participant in his community's cultural activities. They were a major component of his activity and were the focus of much interest and effort—a prime source of positive morale in his life. The freedom to attend cultural activities was to him a major gift of life in the United States (as opposed to the European country where he had been born and from which he had emigrated as a young teenager). It was obvious to everyone who knew him that his ethnic and cultural life was the capstone to his identity. The celebrity status these activities brought to Mr. Meyer was a source of great self-esteem, though his cultural activities were for him an opportunity to discharge his felt obligation to perpetuate his cultural and ethnic heritage.

His wife first noticed that Mr. Meyer was having memory problems after she realized that he no longer looked forward to attending cultural events as he once had. When he would go, he'd participate far less than he had before and reported that while he liked to go, people were "saying nothing new" so he saw no reason to pay attention while at these events.

In spite of a slight recent memory loss, it was felt to be vital to Mr. Meyer's well-being that he continue to enjoy symbolic satisfaction. To the extent that his memory impairment made this less satisfying, Mr. Meyer became somewhat dysphoric. Counseling focused on:

1. Maintaining attendance at cultural events that did not require much active participation and that were enjoyable (as opposed to business meetings);
2. Helping his wife to accept the change in his functioning and in so doing keep her from badgering him to enjoy himself more, remember more, be more sociable, etc.;
3. Keeping cultural media at home so that this avenue of self-actualization could be continuously reinforced;
4. Maintaining social contacts with members of his cultural ethnic community in small groups, preferably at Mr. Meyers's home where greater familiarity and less stimulus competition might minimize anxiety over his poor memory and maximize retention, participation, and enjoyment.

Case Example

Seventy-two-year-old Mr. Weatherwax is a devout Catholic who went to his local church many times a week. His Alzheimer's dementia progressed to the point where he had to take up residence at an intermediate care facility in a neighboring city. This made his usual pattern of religious activity impossible. He confided to his family that he had to go to church but couldn't find one, and that this made him feel sad. The facility, which once had weekly services for its Catholic residents, was unable to find a priest to hold mass on a regular basis. Mr. Weatherwax was asked:

COUNSELOR: Would you like to attend church here in town, or would you prefer to return to your old parish if transportation could be arranged?

CLIENT: Oh, I think I should go where, you know, the people and I know each other. This way they won't think I've left the church.

Transportation was arranged with two of Mr. Weatherwax's old friends who agreed to take him each Sunday to mass at his old church. The family was very grateful as so much of Mr. Weatherwax's life satisfaction came from the observance of his religion. It was a great source of solace and a morale booster through difficult times in his past. In spite of his moderate dementia, this need was clearly expressed and remained a significant activity by which Mr. Weatherwax "found" himself.

Case Example

Dr. Dewey, a retired seventy-three-year-old physician, had mixed-dementia with an eight-year course. He appeared socially well integrated, but could make no decisions on his own, thus requiring vast amounts of time to discuss things with family and care-givers. When not "reading" books (he could not verbalize their content when asked, and his comprehension abilities were suspect when he was seen reading one upside down for an hour), he would play the art critic and deliver long dissertations about the various pictures hanging on the wall. He'd talk about the symbolism, use of color, etc., but his remarks did not validate his claims to be an expert art restorer and critic. His family reported that this was a lifelong pattern, and were interested to see that he was able to preserve a meaningful activity amidst his confusion—his hobby of trying to convince people that he was something he wasn't.

Counseling intervention with Dr. Dewey focused on trying to get him to participate in activity therapy in order to preserve his cognitive and social abilities. His fragile sense of self did not allow him to attempt such a risk, and he preferred to stay detached from those around him. He nevertheless complained that there was nothing to do all day, and that he should therefore be sent home. All suggestions as to what he could do were rejected as being suitable for the other residents, but not appropriate for "a man like me."

The reader is also referred to the description of Molly Gruber in chapter 1, who tells how she used to read and discuss what she'd read with other people. Her apathy toward the recreational programs in the nursing home where she lived was in large part due to the unavailability of recreational activities she found meaningful. In this sense meaning came to denote activities by which Molly could locate herself in her confusion, by the doing of things that evoked a feeling of self-recognition. In the same vein, Dr. Oliver Sacks writes of Jimmy, the "Lost Mariner" who had Korsakoff's syndrome, and was, though he lived in the 1980s, stuck in 1945 as a young man in the navy. Nobody at the nursing home where Jimmy lived could find a meaningful activity for him to replace the roaming that occupied his time each day. Only when somebody observed what Jimmy did, what he found to be meaningful, did it become possible to provide him with opportunities where he found some personal satisfaction.[6]

Case Example

Mrs. Berger is seventy-two-years-old and has had Alzheimer's dementia for about ten years. She recently entered a long-term care facility because she couldn't care for her personal needs and her constant walking made it impossible for her family to care for her. Upon her admission to the facility, she attached herself to Ms. Dorsey, another resident with dementia. The attachment was so strong that Mrs. Berger would not tolerate any separation from Ms. Dorsey, who tried unsuccessfully to go her separate way. Mrs. Berger held on tightly. The two spend much of the day walking around the first floor of the facility holding hands. (Ms. Dorsey has since had trouble maintaining her weight due to all the physical activity she gets.)

Mrs. Berger's family reports that this clinging attachment is a repetition of her reaction when previously institutionalized as a three-year-old girl after her parents divorced. Her father felt that he couldn't care for her properly so, as was the custom of the day, he placed her in an orphanage. There she met and immediately attached to a four-year-old boy, whom she stayed attached to throughout childhood and whom she married when they were in their early twenties. This relationship continued another twelve years until the husband died. Mrs. Berger continued to have serial, dependent, interpersonal relationships with other men, and later with her two sons until she was placed in the facility. Her self-esteem and reduced anxiety level was very much a matter of having another person present at all times.

While both women were intact enough to be counseled about trying to separate from each other during the day, Mrs. Berger would not allow Ms. Dorsey to be separated from her. She became agitated, angry, and frequently struck out at staff when they tried to take Ms. Dorsey away from her. Counseling then shifted to the staff, and discussions were held to develop a plan to keep the pair in one area of the facility and to encourage longer rest periods.

A seldom-discussed component of a demented individual's interpersonal need system is the opportunity for sexual satisfaction. Sexuality is usually discussed only as a problem area because of sexual "acting out" or otherwise-designated sexual misbehavior. Sexuality is, however, a component of the need hierarchy of people with Alzheimer's disease, though opportunities for gratification are typically reduced as part of the process by which behavior becomes disorganized and others withdraw from the patient. Spouses or sexual partners frequently report a loss of libido as a reaction to the stress of care giving, as well as to the aversive responses they feel to the behavioral deterioration of their partner. Physical properties of the patient, such as lack of concern with appearance or cleanliness, contribute to loss of the partner's sexual desire. Finally, the spouse may feel alienated from the person on a sexual level though feelings of love and affection, affiliation and friendship persist and constitute the core of the relationship as physical dependency increases. The patient may express sexual needs but be unable to carry on the couple's previous level of sexual satisfaction. In some cases initiating sexual contact may be evidence of the patient's need for physical closeness, comfort, and reassurance.[7]

Case Example

Mrs. Reardon, a fifty-seven-year-old mother of nine with moderate dementia, was very upset one day and asked to see the consulting psychologist in the long-term care facility where she lived. She was very tearful, so her deteriorated verbal ability made it difficult to understand her concern. Adding to her usual dysfluency was the effect of the discomfort she felt in talking about what bothered her. She wanted to have sexual relations with her husband, she said, but he was rejecting her. One of the unnoticed (by the facility staff) and unsatisfied needs she had was to continue to have sexual expression as part of her marital relationship. Mrs. Reardon's rational and appropriately expressed sexual frustration was very poignant to witness because her normally reticent nature appeared to have been severely stressed by her revelation of this intimate need. She struggled valiantly to make her feelings clear in spite of her inability to finish a sentence consisting of more than four words.

Counseling for Mrs. Reardon's dilemma consisted of a two-tiered intervention. During the first, her risk taking to express her needs was supported and given validation to facilitate more verbal expression and to give some emotional comfort. This was particularly helpful in ameliorating feelings that she would be perceived as crazy or sick because of what she felt she wanted. The second intervention was accomplished by telephone with her husband, who had become very annoyed and asked to speak to someone about the requests for sexual intimacy his wife had been making of him.

MR. REARDON: My wife wants us to have sex! Can you imagine! She can't remember what day it is, or whether I've visited her, but she can remember that she wants sex and she remembers to ask for it when I visit. I've never heard of anything like this.

COUNSELOR: Her feelings for you and her enjoyment of sex are very important ways she has to feel good about herself, to feel attractive and loved. She's a young woman whose self-esteem is being eroded by her disease and the loss of her home, her children, and her normal marital relationship with you.

MR. REARDON: But I don't feel normal. How can you feel normal when your wife is sloppy looking, can't remember to go to the bathroom sometimes, can't take care of the children or the house, and can't hold a conversation. She's like a helpless child. I can't make love to that!

COUNSELOR: I can understand that you feel turned off, and I think the problem should be dealt with directly rather than by avoiding it.

MR. REARDON: Do you suggest I talk to her and tell her all this?

COUNSELOR: I think if you spoke to her and told her that your feelings had changed, and that you loved her and cared for her but weren't able to enjoy sex with her at this point, it might help. At least she could get angry, sad, and grieve the loss of that source of her satisfaction and self-esteem. She might go on to find other ways to feel good about herself as best she can. The program here can help her with that. Would you like a nurse or a counselor to help you by speaking with you more or by having a meeting with you and your wife?

MR. REARDON: Let me think about it. I don't think it would do any good to talk with her.

Mr. Reardon's response was a typical expression of his pessimism and the distancing of himself from his wife and her problems. As his wife became less able to perpetuate her self-esteem in the ways she had prior to her illness, she became more lonely, depressed, and underwent a noticeable personality change as her bereavement continued.

Case Example

Dialogue:

COUNSELOR: Mrs. Ford, how are you, today?

Mrs. Ford: Oh, my name is Miss Brown. I don't know any Mrs. Ford.
Counselor: Were you ever married?
Mrs. Ford: No, I don't think so.
Counselor: *(shows a picture of Mr. Ford, her husband, and their daughters taken six months before)* Do you know this man?
Mrs. Ford: No. Who is he?
Counselor: He's Mr. Ford. Do you know anybody by that name?
Mrs. Ford: No.
Counselor: Do you know any of these three young women? And this man?
Mrs. Ford: No. Who are they?
Counselor: That's you and your daughters, and the man is your husband.
Mrs. Ford: I don't see how that can be. I'm not married. Why would you try to fool me?

The counselor opted not to pursue attempts at reality orientation using photographs, but waited until the family came to visit to do this. She was able to accept their explanation of how they were related when they were present, but could not recognize them in the photos on her dresser. When she was called by her first name, she was able to respond appropriately and appeared to become more relaxed. In this case, the counseling helped Mrs. Ford and those around her connect with an aspect of her "self" that had not yet been erased by receding memory and failing cognition.

One of the more remarkable phenomena care-givers report is how Alzheimer's patients, when allowed freedom of movement (i.e., are not physically restrained) and some freedom of association, are able to form friendships and affiliate with others in their environment. If this need is there and is able to be satisfied, a great deal is contributed to the self-esteem of patients who become known in the present by others who do not know what each one cannot do any longer.

Mrs. O'Brien has moderate dementia. The seventy-seven-year-old former nurse lives in an apartment which is part of her son and daughter-in-law's house. The family is rather dedicated in their attempts to keep Mrs. O'Brien at home in spite of some major difficulties with self-dependence. She will, for example, eat an entire two-pound box of chocolate and then immediately claim that she is never fed, or refuse to allow her son to discard bags of lawn cuttings and leaves. She takes these into the garage when they are left out on the curb to be discarded, and when asked why she does this replies, "You shouldn't throw anything away; you might need this in the future." When asked why this refuse might be needed in the future, she replies, "Oh, I don't know, but somebody will think of something."

Mrs. O'Brien responded to firmly set but quietly and gently communicated limits as to how much she could save.

Sometimes, counselors need to provide reality orientation by expressing a wish that patients not be exposed to danger.

Case Example

COUNSELOR: Mrs. Wright, your husband is upset because you go outside without a coat on when it is very cold. Could you and I agree that you will try to remember to wear a coat each time you go out? NOTE: *(Mrs. Wright is not confronted with her behavior—which she usually denies, but is rather invited to join a joint effort. Her positive feelings for her husband, and hence his concern are also tapped into.)*

MRS. WRIGHT: I never go out without a coat. He worries too much.

COUNSELOR: I am going to ask that you always wear a coat if your husband recommends it. You can help choose which one you'll wear each day.

5

Counselors Have Feelings, Too

Counselors, psychotherapists, and the like are often regarded as perfect paragons of patience, understanding, and wisdom. They are perceived as having no feelings of their own, and as the embodiment of the ideal parent, the wise "father" or all-nurturing mother that all of us wish we'd had. Some counselors unfortunately get caught up in this idealized fictional portrayal and attempt to become this unattainable pedestal dweller.

The more mundane reality is that counselors are human beings who have feelings just like anyone else. These feelings can be the foundation of a considerable source of their ability to provide help and do so in a way that promotes client autonomy. As objective as a counselor tries to be, he/she is still vulnerable to the intrusion of attitudes, biases, emotions, values, and experiences in his/her own past that may color the counseling relationship and can effect its outcome.

Feelings of the Counselor

It is helpful to consider the following points with regard to the feelings of the counselor. Note that these principles could apply to any counselor, not just to those working with the elderly or with Alzheimer's victims. The latter group however does provide some unique challenges to counselors that will be discussed later in this chapter.

1. All human beings, including counselors, have feelings.
2. Feelings are neither good nor bad.
3. It is not unusual to experience feelings during counseling.
4. A counselor who has difficulty accepting his/her own feelings will have problems accepting the feelings of a client.

Case Example

Dr. Melville, an experienced mental health professional in his late fifties was asked to evaluate a demented woman in her early eighties. She was referred by her family physician and brought for the consultation to Dr. Melville's office by her daughter who was around Dr. Melville's age. The mental-status examination revealed marked dementia, and the patient's history indicated a diagnosis of probable Alzheimer's disease. A review of the laboratory medical and neurological exams supported this notion, as they were all essentially negative and gave no indication as to another possible etiology for the gradual decline in the patient's cognitive functioning.

Mrs. Wilson, the patient's daughter, was very clear about the fact that she and her husband were unable to care for her mother anymore, as this would involve sharing their small home with her until the husband's retirement in six months. After that point, they wished to relocate in another part of the country to be near their children and to live in a warmer climate. The daughter recognized that this was a "selfish" decision, but was comfortable with it and appeared firm in her resolve. The mother's dementia was severe enough to warrant twenty-four-hour care, and Mrs. Wilson felt it would be better for her mother to be in a long-term care facility where she could have social stimulation and 'round-the-clock care rather than to have her live at home where she would be socially isolated and at risk due to inadequate community-based services.

Dr. Melville was at this point in his life dealing with the impending placement of his own mother in a nursing home in another city. He had a great deal of difficulty accepting the fact that he had, in his mind, reneged on a contract he had made with his mother many years before that he would never allow her to go into a nursing home. Misjudging Mrs. Wilson's comfort with her decision as cold indifference prompted him to try to persuade her to forget about placement and work more diligently to obtain and coordinate services in the community so that her mother could "obtain the benefits" of living at home. His own strong guilt feelings and unacceptable feelings of having failed his mother made it impossible for him to accept and acknowledge as valid Mrs. Wilson's carefully considered, and reasonable solution to her problem.

5. Trying to hide feelings during counseling can be disturbing to the client.

Dialogue

(At the end of a counseling session)

COUNSELOR: Well, our time is about over for today. Perhaps we can talk more at our next visit about your feelings about your mother's attempt to control your life.

CLIENT: OK, but just let me say one more thing because I'm sure I'll forget it by the next session. (*Goes on to talk three to five more minutes about her controlling mother*)

COUNSELOR: (*Who, by this point, and unknown to the client, is feeling very pressured to end the session because he is running late and, most significantly, is experiencing some strong feelings of his own about being controlled by this client's behavior in a controlling manner much as the client describes her mother. He has many feelings about being in such a position, based on having a father who behaved in a similar controlling way.*) Our time really is up for today, and I think it would be more beneficial if we didn't try to rush through these thoughts and feelings of yours. Perhaps we can spend more time on them in our next session.

CLIENT: Yes, I can see you really want me to leave, because your foot is making a kicking motion like you want to kick me out of here! (*This was a good observation and indeed true!*)

At this point the client had perceived what the counselor was trying to hide, namely, that he was getting uncomfortable for a number of reasons due to his increasing annoyance at being controlled by the client's behavior. Such annoyance is not a sign of an inept counselor; in fact this is a common experience for counselors, psychotherapists, and other service providers. But what is significant about this interaction for our present discussion is that the client got a mixed message, i.e., "I'll listen but I'd like to kick you out of here." Had the counselor been more aware of his feelings at the time he could have responded to his strong feelings and said: "I understand how important it is for you to talk about this, but we don't have any more time right now. If it can't wait until next week, perhaps you'd like to have another session between now and then."

6. Expression of the counselor's feelings without therapeutic benefit to the client imposes a new and unfair relationship on the client.

Incumbent upon counselors is the responsibility not to make *their* feelings the subject of a client's counseling session. The potential for this counter-transference is particularly great when counseling geriatric patients, particular demented patients, and their families, since there can be a tendency to view the patient as a parental figure and his/her children as peers or sibling surrogates from whom support and advice might be obtained. Strong feelings about the aging of one's own parents or one's self can evoke in the counselor the need to achieve emotional equilibrium by appealing for help from a client. This can take the form of soliciting advice, an opinion, or agreement about a choice made by the counselor in a similar circumstance.

In severe cases of counselor stress, strong feelings can be expressed directly by crying, raising one's voice, becoming agitated, or verbally haranguing the client. This is an absolute breakdown of the client-counselor relationship as it has been conceptualized here, and is a sign of acute counselor difficulties. Patients with Alzheimer's disease are not always cooperative and/or willing to follow the accepted rules of office decorum, and they can raise the counselor's stress level after repeated attempts to prevent physical destruction of property or ingesting inedible items have proven futile. Moderate frustration is different than the kind of counselor overreaction being discussed here. The following example illustrates the reaction of a counselor who changed the counseling contract:

> Ms. Wendover was a social worker in a day-treatment program for older adults with dementia. Her own life had been a difficult one, but she had overcome many personal adversities to receive an education and to establish a professional career. She worked very hard and identified emotionally with her clients, often saying to them, "I know how you feel," and meaning it! She was particularly fond of spending time in informal conversation with the mildly impaired clients, and did so with an eye toward having a therapeutic benefit in an informal way. Ms. Wendover had no significant emotional relationships with her peers and spent a great deal of her leisure time doing helping things for others (e.g., her mother, friends, as a volunteer at a local agency,

etc.). One afternoon her supervisor observed that she was crying quite openly to a group of clients who reacted by looking disturbed and bewildered. Some became agitated and began to get upset as well. Others got up and walked anxiously away, looking for another place to sit. The supervisor quite gently and appropriately went over to Ms. Wendover, placed her hands on her shoulders, and suggested that they both go to a more private location to deal with what was happening. Ms. Wendover explained that she had been experiencing problems with money, had been feeling very lonely and sad, and had been quarreling with her mother. As part of the group's informal counseling agenda she had felt it might be helpful to ask their advice about what to do about her troubles, since they were all experienced parents and business people. She allowed as how she was sure that helping her would raise the client's self-esteem.

7. The counselor must be aware of and respect cultural, and socioeconomic factors that influence a client's relative comfort with particular feelings and subjects of counseling.

A counselor working with older persons should think about such clients not only as they are in the present time, but as they were when they were growing up, becoming socialized and developing moral, social, and sexual values. Today's eighty-two-year-old grandmother of twelve was born into a vastly different world than was the counselor who is the age of one of her children or grandchildren. Environmental, historical, socioeconomic, geographic, and other differences are important factors to take into account when trying to understand the origins of behavior, values, and attitudes of elderly clients.

It may be very comfortable for a post-World War II baby boomer, now perhaps a professional counselor, to discuss sexuality, individual autonomy, and serial monogamy. Her grandmother would likely have been less than comfortable thinking about or discussing sexual feelings or patterns of sexual activity, divorce, women fulfilling their individual destinies, etc., with a counselor. The social and sexual revolutions that we witnessed, took part in, or were affected by as society changed around us had varying degrees of influence on the past, present, and coming aggregates of older persons in our society.

Counselors must therefore remember that older persons will vary widely in their willingness to think about, discuss, and try to change attitudes, feelings, and behaviors. It is good to bear in mind the primary axiom of medicine—"First, do no harm" when counseling older persons.

8. The counselor's feelings can provide a valuable clue as to how others in the client's life might respond to the client.

Case Example

Mrs. Williams was a seventy-one-year-old wife of a man with moderate dementia, probably Alzheimer's type. While she was able to take care of her husband and their domestic and financial matters quite well, she came to counseling to get advice on how to get the couple's friends to stay in touch. They were disappearing she said "like rats off a sinking ship," a condition she was sure had been caused by her husband's slow but clearly visible cognitive and psychosocial decline over the preceding three years.

Mr. and Mrs. Williams were interviewed together so that he could be evaluated and their interaction style observed. (It is not unusual for a couple's style to change in a slow and unobserved manner as dementia progresses, producing subtle interpersonal changes and increasing the likelihood of dysfunctional interaction.) Mr. Williams was a very pleasant, retired business executive who was aware of his cognitive difficulties but was not overwhelmingly limited by them. He tried to keep up with things around the house (e.g., yard work, small home-maintenance projects, helping with meal preparation) and could do so reasonably well with his wife's assistance. His successes were occasions of great joy for him, and his failures were taken in stride as opportunities to try again and get it right. Mrs. Williams was a devoted and patient care-giver though she reported that before he "got sick" her husband took care of everything and she never had to worry about all these details as she did now.

As Mrs. Williams talked about how her life had changed since her husband became cognitively impaired, the counselor noticed that she was feeling drowsy and couldn't pay attention as she had before Mrs. Williams began to talk about her feelings. The client continued to talk, and as she did she began to complain that she had never been able to get her husband to listen to her very much before he became demented. Since she didn't want to burden him with her feelings at this point, she had tried to talk to their friends but none of them seemed interested. "They'll tell me about their lives," she said, "but when I begin to talk about mine they suddenly have to leave."

The counselor thought about her own reaction—an escape—and correlated it with the description Mrs. Williams gave of her friends. She realized that Mrs. Williams was feeling helpless, depleted, depressed, and very much in need of emotional support. Her constant complaining was well disguised so as not to appear that she was saying "poor me"—which was indeed her message—and she was arousing feelings of anger and a need to escape in the couple's friends and the counselor. Mrs. Williams was bemoaning her fate and disabling her friends with subtle requests that they meet her dependency needs much as her husband had done but of course could no longer do. The counselor was caught unaware and was not prepared to hear the client's message of extreme helplessness and overwhelming dependency. At the next counseling session, the following dialogue took place:

COUNSELOR: Mrs. Williams, I've been thinking about what you said, about how your friends seem to vanish when you start telling about events in your life now that Mr. Williams has the memory problem. I wonder whether when you describe all that you do for George they might feel like you are asking them for help, and whether this might make them feel awkward.

MRS. WILLIAMS: But I'm not asking for anything. I just want them to know how my time is spent. Maybe if they know how George is doing, they won't be so reluctant to come around. You see, they probably think he's much worse than he really is, and don't know what to say or do when he's around. They're afraid, I think, of what he might do.

COUNSELOR: Sometimes when you describe what you have to do, and how your life has changed since George developed dementia, I got the feeling that you look OK on the outside, but are feeling worried and scared deep down inside. The feelings from deep down inside may be the ones your friends are listening to, rather than the outside message that says, "I feel OK and everything is going well."

Notice that the counselor did not confront the client with how she felt, but rather used her own feelings as data that she correlated with the friends' feelings and her own clinical knowledge of how people in Mrs. Williams's situation might feel. The counselor's insight was also presented in a way that respected Mrs. Williams's need to appear in control of things, and gave the client a way to think about her deeper feelings while preserving her desired social persona and self-esteem. The counselor had correctly understood that Mrs. Williams had a strong need to appear in control of herself and her feelings, and would probably not have achieved any benefit from a harsh, ego-jarring confrontation with her fears around dependency, survival, and her own welfare. In this way, it was possible for her to keep on with her caretaking responsibilities while utilizing her lifelong defenses against unwanted feelings. Were these to be lost at this time, Mrs. Williams could have lost sufficient self-esteem and felt enough guilt and anger that her ability to care for her husband might have deteriorated or ceased.

At a subsequent counseling session, this dialogue took place:

MRS. WILLIAMS: You know I never realized how much I depended on George for everything. He did so many little things without my being aware of them that they seemed to run by themselves. Now that he can't remember what to do or how to do some of them, I see that there was nothing automatic about it.

COUNSELOR: How do you feel about having to do these things?

MRS. WILLIAMS: I'm a bit confused about how to take care of many of them, and I sometimes feel like things will continue to unravel and there will be nothing I can do to stop the process. I realize I probably could do with some help, but I don't know whom to ask. My children all live out of town and I don't want to be a burden to them, or to our friends. They all have their own troubles. Besides, I wonder whether it wouldn't set George back to think that he and I can't go it alone as we did in the past. I worry that he'll get worse if he sees I have to rely on someone other than him.

In this dialogue we see that the counselor's suggestion that the client might have some feelings about dependency not yet able to be expressed openly has been internalized and has produced the beginnings of Mrs. Williams's attempt to explore her feelings about real dependency issues for both Williamses. The counselor was then able to utilize the nine-step counseling model to help Mrs. Williams sort out her feelings and arrange to get her needs met by community resources. She explored her feelings about dependency and its role in her relationship with George, as well as her need to preserve the image of George's autonomy well past his actual ability to do many of the things he had previously managed to do. Mrs. Williams also looked at her own autonomy and capability, and came to understand how she had to overcome her early socialization and allow the development of her own independence and competency in areas of her life where she had been dependent on her husband or others.

This case is an example of how beneficial use can be made of a counselor's feelings in the context of a counseling relationship. Not all interactions work out as well or proceed with such mutual insight, but the potential can be realized in many such cases when given the proper assistance. Telling a person how he/she affects others in a way that preserves self-esteem can be one beneficial outcome of counseling in which the counselor preserves the mutual contract between him/her self and the client, and allows his/her feelings to play a beneficial role for the client.

Clues to Counselor Discomfort

In some instances, feelings may develop in a counselor to the point where an intense personal or intimate relationship is sought with the client. When these feelings arise it will not be possible to maintain the objective position the counselor requires in order that the client's needs be primary, since the counselor now has an emotional stake in the client's life and hence in the outcome of the counseling process.

Complex or chaotic life circumstances of multiproblem older persons or families where dementia is a disruptive factor are not uncommon, and are usually the stimulus for many strong feelings in helpers. It is not unusual for a counselor to feel anger, for example, at the slow pace at which a bureaucracy handles a client's application for benefits or long-term care placement. Similarly, a counselor may experience intense frustration with a family member who is obstructive, negativistic, or dishonest in dealing with a demented relative's care needs. The counselor has a professional responsibility to refrain from expressing angry feelings to a worker at another agency (even though they might possibly be dragging their heels about helping one's client) or at a son whose only involvement in his demented mother's care is to obstruct and/or dismantle a care system that is the result of long, painstaking efforts. Rescue fantasies thrive in such instances, and counselors must refrain from expressing their frustration as anger to such uncooperative persons under the guise of speaking for the client. In actuality it is the counselor's anger that results in the need to be overinvolved, though often not without strenuous encouragement or manipulation by the client.

Helpless feelings brought on by a client's behavior can also produce wishes that the client move away, disappear, die, or become magically better. These feelings are a sign that the counselor feels stuck or immobilized and is angry about it. Since anger toward clients is unacceptable to the counselors self-esteem and not what a "good counselor" feels, the solutions generated in the counselor's mind free him/her of the "no-win client" through circumstances in which the counselor is a victim just as much as the client. When working with Alzheimer's-disease patients a counselor may harbor intense feelings that the diagnosis will be proven wrong and a curable condition found instead, that the client might become significantly worse and require the services of another set of providers (usually a nursing home), or that the patient or family will find it inconvenient to come for assistance and terminate involvement with the counselor.

Counselors who feel like this frequently begin to reschedule these problem clients repeatedly or habitually miss appointments with them. They are unaware of the extra confusion they are causing and do not perceive the message of threatened rejection and abandonment they are giving the client and his/her family. Dementia patients and their families can be very sensitive to feelings of hostility and rejection from others, and may indeed therefore fulfill the counselor's own wish that the client disappear by never returning again.

Complete lack of progress may also signal that the counselor's feelings are a source of interference in the process of providing help. An inability to "hear" the client say important things, or consistently diverting the conversation away from certain emotionally sensitive and therefore uncomfortable subjects are ways in which the counselor's discomfort, and the feelings at the root of it, impede the progress counseling can bring about.

Finally, feelings of fatigue, drowsiness, restlessness, or continually drifting attention may also signify that subjects are being discussed or solutions proposed by a client that arouse strong feelings in the counselor. These reactions are withdrawal or escape devices that enable the counselor to avoid listening to things causing discomfort and threatening to provoke overt displays of emotion. Displays of anger or sarcasm by the counselor are often a sign of similar feelings but are a more overt show of aggression.

What makes these feelings occur in counseling? The answers are varied and based in large part on the individual personality of the counselor and feelings resulting from the counselor's life experiences that leave him/her sensitive to a particular subject or client characteristic(s). That is, there are *counselor variables* and *client variables* that can interact when they meet to produce strong feelings in the counselor, or each can be an underlying source of blocking in counselors due to his/her emotional difficulties in a particular area. A counselor who is experiencing marital difficulties, for example, may unknowingly harbor great anger toward persons of the same gender as the spouse, or see his/her current marital difficulties in most clients' situations. There are other counselor variables that influence work with older demented or depressed clients, and sick or disabled persons, and that can be potential sources of interference to counseling success. These include:

1. Fear of one's own aging.
2. Feelings about the aging of a relative or friend.
3. Fear of incapacitation or severe illness when old.
4. Feelings about one's parents who are ill, incapacitated, or the fear that they will become so.
5. Fear of losing one's mental ability (i.e., "There but for the grace of God go I") triggered by interacting with demented people.
6. Fear that dementia could be transmittable or that the counselor is genetically prone to dementia (especially Alzheimer's type). (This is related to a common fear of "losing one's mind" reinforced by the "myth of senility." People who work with the demented develop a kind of "gallows humor," which is seen when they forget something and will say, "Oh I see I've got early Alzheimer's" or "You see, it *is* contagious.")

7. The anxiety that goes along with an individual's feelings of vulnerability and feelings of helplessness if one loses one's wits. This is particularly true of all people, not just counselors, who rely on their intellect to earn a living and use intellectual defenses (rationalization, intellectualization) to cope with anxiety.
8. Feelings of energy depletion, which depressed individuals can and do trigger, especially those with cognitive impairment.
9. Feelings of frustration and helplessness when interacting with demented older people who are not as facially expressive and whose reduced emotional expression provides fewer of the usual social cues through facial and other gestures.
10. Reminders of old "family contracts" or unfulfilled expectations for which the counselor is held accountable in his/her own mind or in actuality by the family.
11. Annoyance at clients or patients who are not grateful, cooperative, or in many cases unable to articulate what is wrong.
12. Feelings of revulsion or discomfort when confronted with people who are old and physically unattractive.
13. Feelings that older people in general are not able to change because they are rigid, can't learn, won't remember (all myths about normal aging) so counseling is just a "waste of time."
14. Feelings that older people are experiencing problems because of the aging process per se and will, therefore, continue to get worse no matter what a counselor does.
15. Feeling at a disadvantage due to being younger than one's geriatric clients and therefore knowing less than the client. Such a position undermines the counselor's unrealistic need to feel omniscient so as to be able to help.
16. Feelings that older clients are too needy and prefer to be helped rather than learning to help themselves. The truly dependent, needy, clients can frighten a counselor when they become clinging and helpless.

All of these feelings can be triggered by the primary patient, i.e., the demented older person, their older relatives (spouses, in-laws), or their younger or middle-aged children.

Marmor[1] suggests that the origins of strong feelings like these in a therapist (and in a general sense his advice applies to counselors, any helper, or others) arise from two levels of emotional response that are part of any therapeutic interaction. The first, conscious level he terms "appraisal," wherein feelings arise that are appropriate to the objective dimensions of the client. Seeing an older person who is physically healthy and cognitively intact might produce feelings of surprise if a counselor believes that all older persons are chronically ill and confused. Entrance into a nursing home for the first time might cause conscious feelings of fright, revulsion, nausea, or anxiety if the counselor is overwhelmed by the sight, sounds, smells, and other stimuli that can pervade this environment. Trying to interview a confused client who cannot answer a question or sit still for thirty seconds can elicit feelings of frustration or annoyance. The sight of an older person who does not take proper care of his/her physical health, appearance, or personal hygiene can cause a counselor to feel repelled and to become aware of wishes to escape. Interacting with an Alzheimer's patient with mild dementia who denies all cognitive impairment in a hostile suspicious way can make a counselor feel defensive or hurt that the client is not cooperative or trusting. These are some of the many conscious feelings that a counselor might be called upon to process and respond to while interacting with a cross-section of elderly.

On the unconscious level, however, feelings occur in the counselor that are stimulated by the client but which emanate from past significant individuals and situations in the counselor's past. The significant occurrence at this level is that the counselor unwittingly responds emotionally as if the client were another person from his/her past. Thus, for example, a counselor might consciously recognize that a client is being difficult and rejecting attempts at problem solving, but might react with disproportional rage or anger if feelings crop up that remind the counselor of a parent who could never be satisfied by anything the counselor did as a child. Many professionals (physicians, nurses, counselors, clergymen, etc.) report feeling angry when a patient, client, etc., provokes feelings that they are never able to do enough or to do the "right thing." Many are able to pinpoint a person in their life—usually a parent—who gave them the same message when they were children and toward whom they have harbored much unexpressed anger. When helping a client who asks for help and then rejects solutions or assistance, the counselor may feel as if he/she is being told once again that he/she has failed to live up to expectations of highest performance ("You only got a ninety-five? Where are the other five points?"). Unconscious feelings can be triggered in such a way as to be unrelated to the gender, age, or physical appearance of the client. The qualities of the relationship and especially the essential nature of the emotional conflict can be triggered in a counselor or other helper despite concrete dissimilarities between the client and the significant person from the past. The client is a stimulant for dormant emotions.

Client variables are the other contributors to the emotional response of the counselor when interacting with clients. These qualities of the client are experienced at the appraisal or conscious level and are the objective, overt attributes and aspects of the client—in short, the stimuli that arouse the feelings discussed above. A client's gender, age, race, social class, intellect, affect, dress, personality traits, interpersonal style, eagerness to cooperate and achieve counseling goals, and overt attitudes toward the counselor are some of the variables that interact with the counselor's personality, values, and feelings to produce either synergy or dysfunctional blocks in the counselor's mind. The latter typically become clear in consultation with peers or supervisors in case discussions. Productive work with the "difficult client" often resumes after such consultation by the counselor.

Client variables that can evoke strong, unconscious feelings as well as disapproval or negative appraisal can include:

1. A client's lack of physical attractiveness, or a physical disability, disfigurement, or physical presentation (poor grooming, poor hygiene).
2. Communicative impairments such as voice disorders, hearing difficulties, aphasia, articulation disorders, or bilingualism when the client is not as expressive or fluent as the counselor. Dementia patients can typically pose quite a communicative challenge to counselors.
3. Grossly bizarre behavior in an older, confused, or psychiatrically impaired client (e.g., with schizophrenic, bipolar disorders, or depression).
4. Excessive hostility, manipulation, exaggerated helplessness, sexual demands, requests for money, food, and other perceived "violations" of the counseling contract.
5. More comfort or less inhibition by the client about a particular subject than the counselor, e.g., sexuality, death.

6. Sexual disinhibition, urinary or fecal incontinence, verbal or physical assaultiveness, such as seen in dementia patients.
7. Grossly antagonistic behavior by a client or his/her family.
8. Invitations for a "magical rescue." An example of this is the seventy-four-year-old retired musician who was severely depressed with a resulting mild dementia. He pulled up to the counseling center (where he had been receiving counseling and social work services) in a taxicab, unloaded three cardboard boxes, put them in the center lobby, and sent the cab away. He told his counselor, "I know you'll find me another place to live, so I moved out of my room!"
9. "Help-rejecting complainer" clients who proclaim helplessness and then discount or dismiss all suggested solutions or offers of help. This is a manifestation of depression in which the "helpless," angry client is actually exercising passive control over people and getting them to feel angry. The resulting rejection of the client out of frustration reinforces his/her already-considerable feelings of helplessness, isolation and personal unworthiness, and fulfills the client's prophecy that "nobody will help me."

Clients who are demented will present a more complex challenge to counselors, since in addition to any of the above-mentioned traits they may have they are likely also to have trouble expressing themselves, paying attention, following through on a plan or even remembering that any prior meeting(s) took place. Counseling is not wasted on them however, since just participating in such an interaction can provide interpersonal gratification and reinforce the client's sense of worth, self-esteem, and make him/her feel like part of "the team." The memory of having had a "nice talk" with someone, even if the content is gone from memory, can be reassuring to persons with early to middle phases of dementia.

Client variables become multifold and interact with the counselor's feelings in more complex ways when a family system or subsystem is undergoing counseling along with their demented patient. The counselor in this case is dealing with the product of a number of personalities interacting with each other as well as with him/herself. The counselor and client variables at both the *appraisal* and *unconscious* levels are operative for each person in the interaction, and therefore produce many more opportunities for the counselor to experience strong overt feelings and intense covert emotional responses. The behavior of family members counseled in such group settings can turn out to be quite different from what would be the case if each were seen alone or in pairs.

Families that function in a chaotic or otherwise-dysfunctional manner are prime candidates for arousing strong "unprofessional" emotional responses in counselors. Such families often become more chaotic, disorganized, frustrated, helpless, etc., *as a result of* trying to contend with a member who has Alzheimer's dementia or a related disorder. All families that appear so were not necessarily dysfunctional throughout their history, so the counselor may wish to evaluate the degree of stress that Alzheimer's disease has inflicted on the family system in addition to its impact on the patient. (See chapter 3.) Just as Alzheimer's disease can devastate a family, so too can it do great harm to a counselor who felt quite competent until confronted with Alzheimer's disease or another dementia he/she knows little about. Most counselors derive satisfaction from helping clients feel better or solve a problem. Work with demented patients and their families can quickly erode a counselor's self-esteem and sense of professional competence, because the patient does not get well and the family's burden only gets heavier. Closure is temporary since each solution to a problem can be made obsolete by the progress of the dementia. Such experiences "defy our omnipotence (and) rip holes in our omniscience." The clients "constantly threaten to dirty our clean skins, clothing, bill of health, or our medical record of success in treatment."[2]

Nevertheless, counselors can derive positive feelings of success from their work with older, demented clients and their families if they have realistic goals and accept the limitation that the dementias impose on even the most gifted of us. It is helpful to bear in mind that no matter how frustrated, angry, resentful, or defeated the counselor feels, these feelings are limited in duration and pale by comparison to what families, care-givers, and even the patient can feel. These people's feelings are properly the target of counseling intervention since they are the ones who suffer the ravages of Alzheimer's and other dementias.

6

Understanding, Explaining, and Intervening When Problem Behavior Occurs

Mrs. Fleidner calls the police every day and asks them to come get the strange people out of her house. Mr. Marshall is sent out every night by Mrs. Marshall to find the children and bring them home. Mrs. O'Neil packs her belongings daily and sets out for home. Mrs. Taylor's wardrobe grows by a few items every day. Mr. Bloomfield starts to pace up and down at 4 o'clock daily. Mr. Michaels jumps up on the table and engages in attempts at oriental martial arts if anyone comes near him. Miss Reed stops the elevator between floors every day and smiles when asked why.

All of these are examples of some of the problem behaviors that care-givers to dementia patients are constantly called upon to handle with aplomb and patience. They are the very behaviors that cause constant stress, chagrin, anger, despair, and feelings of being overwhelmed and helpless among care-givers. Each family member or other care-giver has his/her own threshold of burden[1] beyond which coping becomes impossible without help.

The most immediate thing counselors can do to provide relief is to inform family members/care-givers that these problem behaviors are not willful or conscious, nor are they vengeful acts of selfishness or laziness. Families should be helped to understand these behaviors are the result of the cognitive deterioration brought on by dementia and as such will not disappear if the appropriate lecture is delivered to induce guilt or remorse. Appeals to reason likewise will not work, since the patient has no control over these behaviors and cannot "act reasonably" when asked.

To help counselors understand these problem behaviors, and thereby help families/care-givers understand them, some of the major behavior difficulties reported by family care-givers[2] are discussed below. If the origins of these behaviors and some intervention strategies can be taught to families/care-givers, perhaps their burden can be lightened, their anxieties reduced, and their efforts reinforced as they cope with these manifestations of dementia every "Thirty-six Hour day."[3]

Wandering

This term is used to describe a group of behaviors that are problems both in home management and institutional care. One definition of wandering is that it is "a tendency to move about, either in a seemingly aimless or disoriented fashion, or in pursuit of an indefinable or unobtainable goal."[4] It is such a problem largely because it occurs at a point during the course of cognitive deterioration when the person is alert, ambulatory, fully conscious, and in good health, but with impaired judgment, spatial disorientation, and abstract thinking ability. The net effect is that the relatively intact physical capabilities of the demented person propel him/her into situations for which he/she lacks the requisite cognitive skills to ensure successful adaptation and appropriate coping.

Wandering can be viewed as a prototypical example of the dysfunctional behaviors that arise from an emotional response to stress in demented persons. It results from the anxiety the person feels as he/she is overwhelmed by a multitude of internal and external stimuli that can not be taken in and processed into meaning rapidly enough to allow the patient to understand things and feel comfortable. Thus, wandering could be characterized as a form of communication[5] by which anxiety is portrayed in nonverbal ways. It may be an especially characteristic adaptation for individuals who have historically been less verbal and less sociable.[6,7] As Hiatt[8] and Snyder et al[9] point out, wandering can be viewed as adaptive or functional for the patient's psychosocial equilibrium because it provides a way of coping with stress and reducing tension. Maladaptive as it appears to be from the care-giver's perspective, wandering and related behavior may represent:

- The patient's lifelong patterns of coping with stress, where the tension generated as a result of finding oneself in a "new," strange environment[10] (whether newly admitted to a nursing home or because once-familiar places are no longer recognized

each day) gets released as it did in the past. Kindred behaviors that were acceptable to others in earlier years include taking a stroll, pacing, fidgeting, or walking while trying to work out a problem.[11]
- Previous work roles, so that industriousness, a formerly adaptive trait is manifested as (1) an identified attempt to continue the same pattern ("I have to take care of my children now"), (2) an unlabeled but clear desire to do so, e.g., rearranging furniture or wiping surfaces with a cloth or hand, or (3) the perpetuating of an old way to the release of energy by attempting to preserve the behaviors of a habitual work role. The behavioral organization, i.e. identifiable patterns to make actions recognizable as a particular task are lacking (e.g., going through the motions of picking up dust or lint), or simply discharging energy in a compulsive way (e.g., pacing) without any identifiable components of a task performed in the past (e.g., sweeping, dusting, mopping).
- A search for security, wherein a person once associated with feelings of security, tension reduction, and lowered anxiety (spouse, parents, sibling) is sought in the "present" although they are no longer alive. Still, they exist in the mind of the patient and are "real" because he/she is living in a present time limited by the receding boundaries of failing recent memory.
- A behavioral way of saying "I feel lost" or "I am looking for things I've lost."[12] Cognitively impaired persons who wander for this reason are searching out familiar landmarks—whether objects, faces, or places by which to locate themselves in time and space. As they lose the ability to scan their memories so as to match images of where they are now with images of familiar places from the past, the search-and-match operation becomes an active physical process rather than a mental one.
- An assertion of the patient's will, autonomy, or last resort taken to sustain one's dignity.[13] This may be especially true of institutionalized patients who may be responding to the homogenizing, regimented, impersonal, atmosphere of the "total institution."[14]
- A response to boredom. Many patients with dementia find themselves in environments that offer few opportunities to do interesting things with any degree of safety. Even in the most loving home situation, there often are not many occasions when a demented person can do something gratifying without being

prohibited from carrying out his/her actions to completion. Otherwise, attempts to do something stimulating usually lead to disasters of varying magnitudes (e.g., cooking the soup until the pot burns, washing ones dirty underwear along with the dishes). Thus, living at home does not guarantee the demented person freedom from boredom, though it may certainly provide feelings of security and familiarity. Chances of becoming bored in an institution are great since there is usually much free time available, and demented people characteristically are not able to structure their leisure time very well. A response to boredom, stimulus seeking frequently prompts demented people to wander in institutions.

- Escape from the overstimulation that patients may experience in a busy home or in an institution that, paradoxically, can be of little interest but filled with aversive disorganizing stimuli such as high noise levels, crowds of (other confused) people, mass activities (like dining and recreation programs), voices on public address systems, etc. These can represent stressful situations for the demented patient who is unable to make sense of these and other complex stimulus environments. The ability to perceive patterns of meaningful vs. nonmeaningful stimuli possessed by the cognitively unimpaired in fact is impaired in many dementia patients. Thus, withdrawal by ambulation, "wandering," is an effective way to reduce the noxious experience of feeling overwhelmed by a flood of stimuli whose pattern and meaning are unclear.
- A response to being lost, and therefore an attempt to find one's way home. Unlike the search for the past that is the basis for some wandering, this variety of wandering occurs when the person recognizes that he/she has lost the way to or from a familiar place.
- A reaction to prolonged use of psychoactive drugs, particularly in veterans of prolonged psychiatric institutionalization. This is, however, a movement disorder and not a manifestation of dementia per se. It may be present in dementia victims who have been on long courses of antipsychotic (neuroleptic) drugs.

Once the care-giver(s) and the counselor have reviewed these possibilities and other possible bases about the cause of wandering, a management strategy can be devised. Remember that wandering is a complex, motivated behavior and will likely take a while to be controlled. Some cases of wandering may be only minimally amenable to change, particularly wandering that is a manifestation of lifelong ways of coping with stress or from internalized work roles.[15] The best one can possibly do with these people is to provide structured, supervised opportunities for the expression of these needs (long walks, folding clothes, etc.). In cases where the environment might be producing wandering, environmental modification to reduce the complexity of stimuli or add meaningful orientation cues can be of help, as can the introduction of opportunities for interesting experiences leading to feelings of mastery with minimal stress.

Rader advocates that care-givers intervene with wandering behavior based on an analysis of the resident's needs and "agenda." She defines agenda behavior as "the planning and behavior which the congitively impaired clients use in an attempt to meet their felt social, emotional or physical needs at a given time. It includes the client's plan of action."[16] By understanding the client's agenda, the underlying need may be met while the overt behavioral manifestation of the need is allowed to pass without comment.

The same patient may wander for a number of different reasons. Being aware of the wanderer's mood can provide good clues about the response that might work the best. Agitated patients may *need* to release their tension and frustration, while placid ones may need a causal approach with redirection. The "happy wanderer" may be exploring or exercising, and may be managed most effectively if the care-giver joins in the mood and the activity.[17]

Verbal interventions are best oriented toward prompting or directing the patient toward the desired behavior rather than prohibiting the undesired one.[18] Thus, when Mrs. Whitehurst heads for the door it is better to say, "Mrs. Whitehurst, stay in the building" or "Come have a glass of juice with me" instead of "Don't go out the door!" The latter command arouses an emotional response to the emotional content of the command as perceived by the listener, and causes the patient to feel belittled. It also taxes the cognitive apparatus of the patient to come up with an alternative behavior at that moment ("If I don't go out of the building, what shall I do?"). Family care-givers can be helped to formulate their communications so that they convey less frustration and/or fewer attempts to control behavior through the use of guilt or other emotional leverage. Communication should impart the most informative message the patient can process and understand ("Come with me to your room. You can put your pajamas on now").

Family care-givers can also be taught to utilize some of the tricks of the trade that professional care-givers have developed over time. One such approach is to observe the patient and get to know when and under what circumstances wandering might be apt to occur. Knowing the history of the patient, his/her past way of handling stress or strange situations, activities he/she utilized to pass leisure time, and typical responses to large groups or solitude are factors the family can integrate into a meaningful appraisal about the possible origins of wandering at a given time. They also can respond to the wandering by distraction and redirective guidance as opposed to confrontation and blocking, though to do so requires that the caretaker might do a great deal of walking him/her self. Structured activity in the home is a necessary part of family care giving, and the family can develop a list of activities that are representative of the patient's interests, hobbies, etc. (thus are aids in orienting the patient to who he/she is) and are within the range of available skills and capabilities the person retains as well. This will prevent wandering to find stimulation. Likewise, giving the patient some autonomy and the opportunity to make choices from among a limited number of options ("Do you want to help me fold the laundry or would you like to watch TV?") support feelings of independence and dignity. Being surrounded by familiar objects, photographs, neighbors, and family help, the patient feels rooted; such rootedness reduces or forestall the chances of feeling lost.

Wandering can be the behavior that brings the demented person's disability to (often unwanted) public notice. Mr. Michaels became well-known to the police department in his small town because they would find him lost and confused every night around eleven o'clock. His wife, who was equally demented, sent him out each evening to "find the children" (actually her young siblings) and he would dutifully obey. Luckily the police force understood and told him that they'd take him home because the children were all at home in bed. By the time he got home, he had forgotten why he was out, but was visibly relieved to be home with his wife. Wandering can also produce the danger of physical injury and even death.[19] Even when it is supervised, some wandering can be detrimental to physical well-being if the wanderer cannot stop and goes continuously until exhaustion sets in. Other wanderers put themselves in jeopardy by utilizing more calories in a day than they can ingest, and eventually need to be fed while they walk. These patients do especially poorly when restrained and end up becoming agitated, calling out until they are hoarse, getting out of restraints, and injuring themselves by head banging or in their attempts to free themselves from restraints. Such patients are very difficult if not impossible to manage at home and often require institutional placement with continuous assistance by an aide who walks with the patient or a group of staff who can monitor his/her whereabouts.

Agitation

This term is usually applied to a broad category of behaviors ranging from the physical symptoms of chronic neurotic anxiety or affective disorders[20] to some of the problematic disturbances in dementia that stress care-givers to their limits. In dementia, agitation is a behavioral problem akin to wandering but seems to be composed of elements that caretakers, family, and others who live in close proximity to the behaviorally disturbed individual find very annoying and wearing on their patience. Two recent discussions of agitation by Cohen-Mansfield and Billig[21] and by Cohen-Mansfield[22] provide systematic analyses of these behaviors that are helpful from both definitional and conceptual perspectives. Agitated behavior is inappropriate behavior (as judged from the perspective of the observer) that can be manifested as (1) abuse/aggression toward the self or others (e.g., cursing, screaming, yelling at others, hitting, scratching, spitting, grabbing people); (2) appropriate behavior performed to excess (e.g., constant questioning, accusativeness, requests for help, repetition of sounds, words, phrases, or sentences, repetitious mannerisms, constant talking [often termed "verbal incontinence"], pacing, and aimless ambulation); and (3) acts inappropriate to social standards for a given situation (e.g., layering of clothes, disrobing in public places, making strange noises). Agitated behavior of congitively impaired nursing-home residents has been described as comprised of aggressive-physical (hitting, biting, etc.), aggressive-verbal (cursing, yelling), and nonaggressive (pacing, disrobing, dressing in layers).[23]

If there is no evident physical basis for agitation (e.g., pain, fecal impaction, side effects of psychotropic medication, metabolic disorders, nutritional deficits, neurological disorders) then the care-giver/ family member and the counselor can begin to try to understand why the behavior has occurred. As with wandering, it is often helpful to look for the origins of these behaviors in some environmental element that raises the patient's anxiety level to the point of extreme discomfort—a state manifested by the behavioral disorganization that is expressed as agitation. Professional care-givers were asked why they thought patients became agitated, and their observations are very useful in helping us develop hypotheses as to why agitation happens to a given patient. The results of one such investigation[24] indicated that there are a number of interrelated possibilities. These are (1) agitation occurs as a response to an unmet need or as a manifestation or behavioral communication of a patient's mood (depression, loneliness, boredom); (2) agitation is a response to events in the environment, (e.g., other residents' anxiety, incessant talking, rummaging in their room, etc.) or care interventions that are not a good match[25,26] to the patient's temperament or mood at a given time (e.g., being forced to shower or eat at a certain time, being approached too closely or too forcefully); (3) agitation is a disability-based, unsuccessful attempt at or outcome of self-care (e.g., feeding, toileting, dressing, communication); or (4) agitation results when past issues or events have left an emotional residue or afterimage. Even though the actual event itself may have been forgotten (e.g., being spoken to harshly by a caretaker, losing something or someone and feeling discontented until it is found, which is perhaps an impossibility in the case of a dead relative, former home, or imagined possession), the internal feeling state lingers.

Just as in the case of wandering, prevention of future episodes is one of the most effective interventions for agitation, since no amount of punishment or reasoning with the patients will decrease the likelihood of it happening again. (These responses may in fact become more likely after such treatment.) Alertness to mood changes, signs of increasing restlessness and frustration, (louder tone and higher pitch of voice, increased pacing, a "cloud" hanging over the patient, tensed facial muscles, fist clenching) can signal the care-giver that something is brewing in the patient. A soothing tone of voice, smiling face, and easy, slow movements can help to change the patient's mood. Sitting or walking with the patient while inquiring (not interrogating) about what might be bothering him/her can help the patient with remaining linguistic ability begin to try to articulate what might be troubling him/her. Care-givers may have to help the patient articulate the difficulty, source of upset, or feeling by clarifying communication and/or supplying words or phrases where needed. (See "Communicating with Demented Persons" for hints on this topic.)

A care-giver can analyze the sequence of events leading up to the onset of agitation to see whether miscalculations in his/her caretaking behavior may have triggered the agitation. Counselors can prove very beneficial to both family and professional care-givers in this context by teaching them how to reconstruct the chain of behavior as objectively as possible. The "what, when, and how" of behavior can be pieced together, while the "why" is reconstructed from hypothesis about the behavior's origins and not presumed by the caregiver based on his/her own emotional state or interpretation ("He did it to get back at me" or "She's just faking so that I'll take care of her").

Environmental modifications are worthwhile considering if it appears that overstimulation, physical barriers, or distractions, difficulty using the toilet or managing clothing, or the need to escape stimulus overload might be at the root of agitation. Some agitation is quite resistant to intervention and is often best dealt with by hoping to reduce it rather than eliminating it totally. The use of psychotropic drugs to eliminate agitation is not a panacea, as they can cause serious side effects (including oversedation and gait disturbances, falls and lethargy, movement disorders, and increased agitation). Behavioral intervention, along with better management and care strategies can be effective in the long run. Psychotropic medication given under strict medical supervision, with frequent review, and as part of an interdisciplinary approach of appropriate care given can be a useful approach in cases of severe agitation. Finally, it is vital to remember that agitation can be the patient's way of telling the caretaker that something physical, as well as emotional could be the matter. Demented patients frequently lose the ability to identify the location of pain or discomfort (due to an impaired body sense) and frequently respond to physical problems (e.g., stomach pain, elevated temperature) by becoming agitated. This nonverbal signal should be explored and an underlying physical cause ruled out before medications, environmental or behavioral interventions are attempted. Counselors can advise family members/care-givers about these interventions and considerations as to the etiology of agitation. Their efforts at assessing the cause, perhaps with appropriate consultation from other professionals can be discussed, evaluated, and reinforced in the counseling setting.

Catastrophic Reactions

These are a special case of agitation and can be viewed as a sign of complete system overload and cognitive failure.[27] Catastrophic reactions were reported to be a problem by eighty-nine percent of families reporting the occurrence of that behavior. Next to memory disturbance, they were the most reported problematic behaviors.[28] Gwyther[29] describes catastrophic reactions as consisting of sudden change in mood, uncontrollable crying for long periods of time, combativeness, anger, or increased suspiciousness, stubbornness, and worry or tension. These symptoms may occur alone or in combination. A catastrophic reaction can also appear to be like a temper tantrum or fit of rage in a formerly calm adult who is reacting in a disproportionate way to an environmental incident. Some causes for such a reaction can include: being asked several questions in succession (especially *why* questions), feeling lost, left behind, or insecure; being surrounded by many strange people or stimuli (e.g., at a birthday party or family event filled with the "strangers" the patient fails to recognize as family or friends); seeing television shows depicting events the patient has trouble separating from reality and assumes his/her life or relatives are affected by what was seen; being scolded, argued with, or contradicted; caretakers' impatience, irritation, tension or accelerated pace of activity, and failure to perform successfully tasks that used to be routinely completed with ease (e.g., cooking, washing dishes, putting on a pair of trousers).[30]

Catastrophic reactions occur when too many or too complex a series of stimuli cause increased confusion. The frontal lobe, the part of the brain that inhibits the expression of impulses such as anger, rage, tearfulness, or striking out, is frequently deteriorated in Alzheimer's dementia, rendering the patient unable to control the impulses that arise in response to a felt frustration or threat. The patient may also lose the ability to exercise adult judgment about the seriousness of an incident, and therefore is unable to think about how others will feel about his/her behavior. The reaction is thus impulsive, based on exaggerated feelings about the seriousness of the incident and happens without any concern about how others will feel. In these ways it is "childlike" because it represents a developmentally earlier form of thinking and social perception called "egocentric thought," in which the young child is *unable* to see the world from a perspective other than his/her own.[31] Like the young child who has not progressed to the point of being able to imagine what someone else would perceive, feel, think, etc., the demented person who behaves egocentrically (in catastrophic reactions and in other instances as well) is not *choosing* to be self-centered or selfish. He/she is rather a victim of cognitive limitations that result from the product of organic damage and stress working together to reduce the patient's adaptational ability at that moment.

In the event of catastrophic reactions Gwyther recommends: (1) reducing the number and complexity of stimuli in the environment by eliminating noises, and rephrasing questions to make them answerable (reduce the number of choices offered, or asking yes or no questions); (2) giving directions one step at a time in sequence; (3) distracting gradually with a new objective and letting the catastrophic reaction and its precipitant fade into the (forgotten) past; (4) using soothing voice tones during the episode and soothing actions after it is over (stroking the arm, holding hands, rocking to calm the upset patient; (5) NOT RESTRAINING or otherwise putting your hands on the patient while a catastrophic reaction is taking place, as it will probably increase the intesity of the reaction by adding another stimulus to an already-overloaded mental apparatus; (6) moving slowly and narrating your actions as you proceed to intervene ("I'm going to come around to the front of you and button your shirt"); and (7) allowing the memory impairment to work for the maintenance of the patient's self-esteem by not discussing the incident or seeking clarification from the patient as to why the catastrophic reaction took place. Families and other care-givers can be counseled to utilize these approaches and to practice prevention by alerting all other care-givers as to which events or persons in the patient's environment seem to be causing catastrophic reactions. One preventable intervention of great value is to provide counseling opportunities for care-givers/family members so that their pent-up anger does not get discharged when they respond to a catastrophic reaction. Overwhelmed family members/care-givers are, like the patient vulnerable to overload; they may respond with impulsive, emotional expressions of anger that do not take the patient's feelings into account. These will only serve to frustrate or frighten the patient, escalate the conflict, perhaps perpetuate the catastrophe, and make the care-giver feel guilty. Encourage families not to dwell on the day's or week's catastrophic reactions when speaking with other relatives or care-givers, especially when the patient is within hearing range. Nothing discourages contact with the patient like the fear of hearing about or being a witness to catastrophic reactions.[32]

Inappropriate Sexual Behavior

This category of behavior is mostly comprised of three kinds of "inappropriate" actions by the patient. These are (1) exposure of the sexual organs and/or fondling of the genitals; (2) undressing in public view or dressing so that some parts of the body are not appropriately covered (i.e., wearing underwear with no trousers or skirt); and (3) making sexually suggestive remarks or initiating physical, sexual approaches (touching the breast or buttocks) toward caregivers. Sexual behavior towards the spouse is not considered inappropriate in this context since it represents the maintenance of a prior element in the relationship. The spouse may feel uninterested in or uncomfortable continuing a sexual relationship with a person who has changed so drastically and become so unlike him/herself prior to being cognitively impaired,[33] but the patient's interest in sex is not pathological. This discussion will therefore focus on the three behaviors noted above, while the important topic of sexual expression is discussed in chapter 2, "Separation and Loss in Alzheimer's Disease: The Impact on the Family."

First and foremost to consider is the finding that sexually inappropriate behavior is more of a myth than a reality about demented patients.[34] Our society's overall conflict about sexuality, and its anxiety over sexuality in older persons, creates the fertile ground where myths like "the dirty old man" and "sexuality in the aging is a sign of pathology" flourish. An extension of these myths is the fear that "senile" old people behave in sexually deviant ways, a fear that serves to bias the perception of observers as to the motivation and causes of "sexually inappropriate behavior" in the demented elderly. As we shall see, these behaviors are far from being expressions of lust turned loose by the malevolent urges of confused oldsters who wish to molest others or to display themselves sexually. They are, rather, manifestations of confusion with more benign origins though with physical manifestations variably related to actual sexual expression. They are also apparently rare experiences for family care-givers.[35]

Exposing the Genitals and Self-stimulation

Case Examples

Mr. Thompson gets up out of his chair, unzips his pants, and begins to pace the floor while holding on to his penis in full view of everyone in the room.

Mr. Gifford sits in front of the television and rubs his crotch repeatedly. His care-giver finds him with the front of his pants drenched.

These two men are showing typical behavior of demented persons who have the urge to urinate, but cannot recall the appropriate sequence of behavior that they have learned as children in response to that urge. Mr. Thompson gets up to find the bathroom but cannot remember where it is, all the while having begun to do what he would formerly have done when he reached the bathroom. It appears as if he must physically remind himself of what he set out to do by maintaining the physical prompting he needs to keep his behavior goal directed, since his memory of the urge to urinate and the directions his brain may have given him in response to the urge are fleeting.

Mr. Gifford senses discomfort but isn't able to identify the specific message his body is sending his brain, i.e., that his bladder is full and that it requires emptying. He is able to make an attempt to alleviate the discomfort by rubbing the area where he feels the stimulation, but he cannot respond as he once could in order to adapt and empty his bladder in the appropriate way.

In neither of these two cases was the behavior primarily sexual in nature or origin, though because of anatomical realities it could be misinterpreted that the behavioral expression of the confusion felt by the patient because he had the urge to urinate but could not find the toilet was sexual.

Case Example

Mrs. Rose is sitting with her family and proceeds to stand up, hike her dress up to her waist, and walk around looking each person in the eye. Others can see that she is not wearing underpants and is entirely exposed.

Just like Mr. Thompson, Mrs. Rose has an urge to go to the toilet but is unable to act appropriately in response to it. Her self-exposure is an accidental result of having forgotten to put on her underpants that morning. She hiked her dress up in preparation for sitting on the toilet, but couldn't remember what else to do. Her behavior was "designed" to signal her needs to others, since she couldn't articulate her problem in words. Staring at each person was her best available attempt to elicit their attention without making a public spectacle of herself. Because of her impaired social sense, she could not behave in the totally discreet manner she attempted to portray by "catching someone's eye."

The best response to these behaviors is usually (and without over-reaction) to lead the person to the bathroom quietly and say to any one present, "He/she forgets what to do when he/she has to go to the toilet." This will be enough to prevent the behavior from being interpreted in a sexual context and label it for what it truly is.

Demented persons will occasionally engage in masturbatory behavior in full view of others. This is done in response to the brain's command that pleasure be sought. But the portion of the brain that inhibits or postpones these impulses is no longer able to function as it once did, so the command is obeyed immediately. Masturbation, when engaged in by a person of any age elicits strong negative reactions in our culture, so it is not surprising that families and caregivers become very upset when it happens. Counselors can reassure them by explaining why it happens and informing them that it is not a sign that other sexually uninhibited behavior will necessarily follow. Feelings of embarrassment or revulsion may also require discussion. Family members respond well to intervention, which allows them their feelings but puts the behavior into realistic perspective by providing an explanation about its origins. Families can also be encouraged to respond to masturbatory behavior of their demented relative by calmly and gently attempting to redirect the person's activity through distraction ("Let's go into the other room" or "Would you hold onto this string of beads for me?") rather than by becoming upset. Outbursts of anger, moralizing attempts to induce shame or guilt, or rough physical handling are likely to produce angry and even combative responses from the patient and possibly may also trigger catastrophic reactions.

Public Undressing or Incomplete Dressing

Patients with Alzheimer's disease may fidget with buttons until they have opened their entire shirt or blouse, disrobe partially or completely in the middle of the day even if someone else is around, or walk around with their underclothes on top of their shirt but with no pants or underpants on. All of these behaviors are indications that the patient is experiencing some difficulty due to impaired cognition, not signs that he/she is an exhibitionist or sexually perverse.

Total or partial disrobing usually occurs because the person is uncomfortable (too hot or cold, clothes too tight) in what he/she is wearing and cannot identify which item of clothing is the offending one—so all of the clothing must go. Sometimes the patient thinks the clothes he/she has on are not his/hers since they can't be recognized because they are not remembered, and so he/she decides to take them off. The person can be disoriented to time of day and believe it is time to get ready for bed, take a bath, etc., so he/she disrobes when the impulse strikes. The decline of social judgment that demented persons experience is the crucial disability at work here since it permits the patients to go ahead and respond to an impulse regardless of the social setting. At more advanced stages of dementia the person may forget why it is important to be dressed since his/her outlook and internal value system seem to lack feelings of shame or modesty. Dressing is a social convention, after all, and the patient loses awareness of the "self" in a society of others (a kind of egocentric thinking). Empathy and seeing things objectively is too complex a task for impaired cognition.

Making Suggestive Remarks or Being Sexually Aggressive

Many more instances of these behaviors are reported by professional care-givers than by family members, and these usually take place in situations involving the giving of physical care such as bathing, dressing, or other personal care. A demented person who is sexually stimulated as a result of being touched, cleaned, washed, etc., lacks the social judgment and cognitive ability to understand that any physical contact is happening in the context of his/her being cared for and that the interaction is not sexual in purpose. The patient responds exclusively and impulsively to the pleasure of the physical sensation, and, since this is misinterpreted as a message of sexual invitation (this is almost always reported about males cared for by women care-givers), reacts to it in kind by engaging in sexual touching. The patient does not remember his relationship with the caregiver (or relative, for that matter) and may have frontal lobe damage, and therefore cannot be inhibited by taboos, feelings of propriety, or other cognitive barriers to expressing sexual impulses.

Counselors may be called upon to help families and other caregivers understand the origins of this behavior and put it in proper perspective. Intervention should be in the form of simple commands telling the patient what to do and orienting him/her to the activity taking place. ("Mr. Jones, please don't touch me there. I'm giving you a bath. Hold the soap [towel, etc.] while I wash your back.") Giving the patient something to do with his hands is a helpful intervention and a prevention strategy worth remembering. Under no circumstances should this or any other such behavior be discussed in a way that holds the patient up to ridicule or tries to provoke shameful and guilty reactions in the patient or family. It is difficult enough to live with the reality of having a demented relative without having to contend with the stress of being told that he/she is a "dirty old person." Remember that the patient who demonstrates sexually inappropriate behavior does so because he/she has brain damage, and that not every Alzheimer's patient will behave this way. Some patients experience a loss of sexual urges, and some show a marked increase. No matter which response occurs it does not indicate the moral level of the patient or the family.

Sexually Inappropriate Behavior around Children

If any of the behaviors discussed occurs in front of children, families should be counseled to understand that a matter-of-fact, calm response will prevent the situation from becoming overly traumatic for the child. Should the patient be observed in a state of undress, fondling him/herself, exposing his/her genitals or otherwise behaving inappropriately, the adult should quietly remove the patient and explain to the child that the patient forgets how to behave or "forgets where he is."[36] A family prepared through reading or counseling will provide a great deal of preventive intervention if the patient's behavior is explained to the child in such a way that it can be understood as a response to confusion about having to go to the toilet, not liking the clothes he was wearing or "playing with his buttons while he forgets what he is doing," rather than as the sexual behavior of a "dirty old man." Children copy adult's attitudes about these matters, so it is important that grandfather (or Aunt Mary) be treated as an object of respect and understanding rather than as an object of disgust, scorn, and contempt.

Rummaging, Hoarding, and Losing Things

Case Example

Mrs. Fleming lives with her adult daughter because she has a diagnosis of Alzheimer's disease and cannot care for herself. She goes through her daughter's closet every day and "retrieves" blouses, slacks, dresses, shoes, etc., that she insists belong to her and believes that her daughter borrowed without her permission. The daugher gets very upset, since a good portion of her wardrobe now hangs in her mother's closet and no amount of reasoning can change her mother's mind. All of the daughter's attempts to convince her mother that the clothes could not be hers (the size is too large, "here is a picture of me in that dress," etc.) fall on deaf ears and are countered with "Those are mine" from Mrs. Fleming.

Mrs. Fleming's dementia results in her losing clothing daily since she isn't able to remember or recognize them from one day to the next. Since she has no insight into the fact that she forgets which clothes are hers, her mind proposes another explanation of their disappearance—somebody must be taking them! Proof of this hunch is found in the daughter's closet, which contains clothing that must be hers since that is where the disappearing clothes must be kept by the thief. Anything in Mrs. Flemming's own closet is a stranger's, and not hers. The logic Mrs. Fleming uses to explain the case of the disappearing clothing is airtight, and like all closed logical systems, is not penetrable by outside assumptions (e.g., "You've forgotten that the clothes in your closet are yours" or "These things don't fit you, they're four sizes too large"). Her basic assumptions are oriented toward explaining the fact that her clothes "disappear" in a manner that excludes her memory loss as a possible cause. This is totally plausible to her because she does not acknowledge the memory loss at all, and projects blame for her cognitive failings onto others.

Patients with Alzheimer's disease are frequently aware at some level of being conscious that things are "missing," that the world has taken on a different look. But they cannot always articulate *what* is missing. Patients are frequently aware that much has vanished from their lives as their recent memory recedes but cannot formulate this thought in reflective existential terms. Instead, they express these losses (friends, family, home, skills, words, memories, parts of the self) in concrete terms. The feeling that something is lost is correct, but what is lost is not clear or is inaccurately identified. Expressions such as "my belongings are missing" or "somebody took my clothes" are used when the patient cannot otherwise explain how once-familiar items are gone, either because they are not recognized or because they have been (mis)placed in now-forgotten hideaways. (See the upcoming discussion of Hoarding.) Finally, patients are not always wrong or misinterpreting when they report that something is missing. Unfortunate instances do occur when care-givers take things from demented patients, believing "She'll never miss it. She probably can't remember she had that sweater anyway." Any reasonable claim that something is missing from the environment of a demented person should be investigated.

Some rummaging may be explainable as an attempt at orientation. That is, the patient is searching for his/her things in all these strange, unfamiliar locations. Attempts to find familiar objects are, in the words of one patient, ways to be "looking for myself."

Case Example

Mr. Benjamin became quite demented and required placement for his own safety. His family felt guilty and conflicted over this decision, but realized that as neither of his children lived in circumstances that enabled them to care for him, they had no realistic alternative. Their feelings were further disturbed when they received a phone call from the social worker at the nursing home into which Mr. Benjamin had gone saying that he was going into other people's rooms and searching through their dressers and closets and stealing others' belongings. The family attended a case conference at the nursing home the next week and were shocked to be told that a psychiatrist had diagnosed their father as having kleptomania and that he was to be given haloperidol, a strong neuroleptic drug, to control his behavior. The family told the nursing-home staff that Mr. Benjamin was a lifelong, inveterate collector of odds and ends. He would tinker with his gleanings or would save them for a rainy day. They were told that his stealing would have to stop, and that the nursing home would have to restrain him physically if the family was unable to persuade him "to stop stealing."

This unfortunate case example illustrates some counterproductive ways to deal with rummaging behavior, and is also an example of how lifelong traits that were adaptive for the patient become liabilities when dementia (and institutionalization) occur. Mr. Benjamin's family was aware of the origins of his rummaging and understood that it was an expression of his lifelong method of keeping himself busy, rather than an antisocial tendency (kleptomania). The problem at this point in Mr. Benjamin's life was that his impaired cognition rendered him unable to distinguish the difference between junk that people had discarded, his own belongings, and the possessions of other people that were inappropriate for him to search through (an act he had never committed until after he became demented and lived in an institution). Giving Mr. Benjamin a "rummaging drawer" or barrel with a collection of odds and ends or other recreational, structured things to do to keep busy would possibly have curtailed some of his behavior. The erroneous labeling of his rummaging was inaccurate and a further source of hurt to his family. Intervention and counseling should have been oriented toward diverting the behavior into an acceptable environment and securing the places Mr. Benjamin should stay out of. Families should never be made to contend with the pain of such a mislabeling of behavior.

Hoarding

It is not unusual for dementia patients to collect things like silverware, milk cartons, paper napkins, old tissues, coins, shoes and socks, scraps of paper, or other people's dentures. More often than not the "collector" will establish hiding places and quickly forget these "safes," or will place things for safekeeping in locations that are remembered from the remote past. Some favorite places are under a mattress or sofa cushion, in a bureau drawer, in the cupboard or refrigerator if the person cannot distinguish among storage places in the kitchen, etc. Asking the person why he/she does this or challenging him/her to define "why" an old tissue is worth saving will probably elicit an answer like "I might need this" or "You never know when someone might be looking for one." Worse, such inquiries can provoke anger or catastrophic reactions. It is likewise futile to ask a patient where he/she hid the things he/she took since he/she probably can't remember.

There is no single answer to explain the origins of hoarding. It may be a manifestation of lifelong personality tendencies, an attempt to make up for all of the losses the patient has experienced as cognition worsened, or it may be a manifestation of boredom and/or a sign of stress. Some demented patients hoard because their memories have rolled back to the time of the Great Depression or other period of poverty and scarcity during their younger days. They therefore repeat those actions supported by the context of those memories, when one saved everything for potential use in the future. Collecting useful and useless items might appear to be strange behavior, but the demented person's ability to judge from among things that are (potentially) useful or not would seem to be a function of cognitive ability as well as idiosyncratic tendencies, and probably rooted in personal history.

Losing Things

The short-term memory deficit in Alzheimer's disease makes losing things a likely occurrence. The patient who loses things may have forgotten where something was left or may not remember having had the item at all. Some patients will admit to the possibility of their having forgotten where they put something, while others utilize projection or denial as ways of defending against the anxiety they feel when confronted with their behavior. The latter patient might say he/she never had the item in question and that someone else probably lost it, or that it was stolen. The former might say that his/her son, caretaker, etc., took it. As was discussed above, patients will frequently say that something is "lost" when they have misplaced it, or when they have become aware that an item or personal belonging in *their* present reality (i.e., the past, to us) is missing. So, for example, a demented patient may complain with great distress that his/her child is missing or that his/her school clothing is gone. Reassurance and orientation ("Your child is fine. He's at home.") work well when used consistently.

How to Help Families and Care-givers

The counselor who is aware of how and why rummaging, hoarding, and losing things occur can help the family or care-giver troubled by these behaviors in a number of ways. First, the counselor can help by redefining these behaviors as manifestations of cognitive impairment rather than as signs of moral degeneracy. Families/care-givers are better able to follow through on intervention techniques if they approach behavioral difficulties as results of brain damage, rather than if they ascribe other motives to the behavior. Second, counselors can assist family members/care-givers with the practical strategies of preventive care, the most effective long-range intervention for these behaviors. Suggestions can be offered to the family/care-giver to: (1) learn the person's hiding places; (2) secure closets, bureau drawers, etc., with difficult-to-see safety locks, hasps, or other mechanisms so that the patient will not notice their placement, (like placing locks near the floor); (3) provide items a person *can* rummage through if this behavior is needed by the patient; (4) avoid arguments about the actual ownership of a "collected" item not belonging to the patient and quietly removing it from the patient's room or closet when he/she is not present (this may have to be done daily for a period of weeks or more); (5) NEVER call the person a kleptomaniac, thief, or liar; and (6) remove valuable items, such as jewelry, fine silverware, money, etc., from where they might be normally kept and easily found by a rummaging patient. Mace and Rabins[37] further suggest that small items like keys, eyeglasses, hearing aids, and batteries, etc., be kept in duplicate in safe places, and that wastebaskets be checked before their contents are thrown out. Families should also be encouraged to inquire of all family members, especially siblings and age-peers of the patient, about the location of the patient's favorite or traditional hiding places when he/she was young. These might be a good place to begin looking for those vanished objects. Finally, it is good to advise families that those older persons who lived through the Great Depression have very strong and deep memories about the fear and reality of never having enough. They therefore save everything (just as they did during the Depression and World Wars) as they become aware that things are becoming scarce (i.e., they are "losing" them to poor memory). One demented patient when asked why she saved everything told me that she saved thread, sticks, newspapers, and small pieces of scrap (her garage was full of these to the point that her family feared a fire) because "if you lived through the times I did you'd know why I do!"

Suspiciousness, False Ideas, Delusions, and Hallucinations

Loss of memory can make one very anxious, and these often-unacceptable levels of anxiety find expression in various ways. Patients use various defense mechanisms and cognitive operations to make sense of the events occurring around them. These "explanations" may be full of feelings of suspiciousness, persecution, grandiosity, and other signs that the patient's ability to "fill in the gaps" between reality and what his/her mind can comprehend is colored by anxiety and fear. These mechanisms are very troublesome for caregivers and family members, but are very good protection for the fragile self-esteem of the patient. If something is lost or misplaced, it is easier to blame someone else than to blame yourself. (Think about the last time you misplaced your car keys and asked a person you lived with, "Where did you put my keys?") As the patient recognizes fewer people and places in his/her environment, things take on a foreign, "out of place" cast and anxiety builds up. Pressured by anxiety, fears for one's safety, and feelings of being "out of place" and surrounded by strangers, people are more prone to see any problems as coming from outside the self and due to the deeds of others, rather than rising from shortcoming of one's own. In this way the fault for memory loss and its effects—vanished objects, missing people, strange rooms, or clothes—is placed outside the self. The "others" who are blamed are often the very devoted caretakers who react with feelings of hurt, shock, betrayal, or anger.

It is not difficult to understand how people with dementia begin to think in suspicious ways as they experience the losses, mysteries, and newness of life's events each day that result from fading memory. Nevertheless, these behaviors can create marked discomfort in family members/care-givers because they are considered signs of insanity. Families/care-givers can be helped by counselors to understand why these phenomena occur and how best to minimize the disruptions they can cause. Some patients will for example lock the doors, barricade themselves inside a room, call the police, or similarly respond to feelings of being threatened by imagined malevolent persons. Others will experience pleasant perceptions or have positive suspicions, such as Mrs. Black's seeing a puppy dog at the foot of her bed and reporting that she felt "comforted," or Mrs. Stanley's belief that Sammy Davis, Jr., came in through her window to take her to a picnic every Sunday when the weather was pleasant. All of these phenomena may frighten families and care-givers who can benefit from counseling about the nature of such behavior and appropriate responses to it.

Misinterpretations

These behavior problems stem from the congitively impaired person's inability to correlate partial information with logical explanations about the cause of events in the environment. Sometimes the problem lies in the impaired hearing or vision of the patient who misinterprets unclear visual or auditory images and, in the presence of some anxiety, mistakenly construes these to be people doing threatening things (hiding behind the door) or talking about the patient. Suspiciousness exacerbates any tendencies toward such misinterpretations, and increases the patient's feelings of threat or danger in response to the mistakenly understood environmental event.

Families/care-givers can be helped to understand that these are not hallucinations but rather constitute misunderstanding of an event. This is important to many family members because: (1) many institutionalized Alzheimer's-disease patients are incorrectly reported to be hallucinating and given strong psychoactive medicines when they could benefit from other interventions with fewer side effects and (2) families become frightened and may withdraw from the patient or rush to seek nursing-home placement because they fear an escalation of the "crazy" behavior. It is often useful to point out that the visual and/or auditory impairments older Alzheimer's patients may have can help produce these events and that they are often responsive to change in eye-wear prescriptions, improved lighting, rearranging of furniture in the room, or a hearing evaluation or hearing-aid maintenance (are the batteries working?). If a hearing loss is suspected, speakers should be instructed to look directly at the patient, speak slowly and clearly, and include the patient in the conversation when talking in front of him/her. If there are competing sounds in the background that interfere with the patient's ability to understand (due to the problem of paying attention that a demented person may have), or if voices on the television are not loud enough, adjustments should be made to reduce the excess disability[38] and decrease chances for misinterpretations to occur.

Some misinterpretations occur because of environmental features that play tricks on the patient's eyes or ears. The patient may report that someone is spilling water or putting ice in his/her room because of mistaking the shiny finish on a tile or linoleum floor as being wet or icy. This is due to the reduced acuity of the older eye, which does not see well when glare is present. (To visualize this misinterpretation, take a look at a polished floor with a high shine when the sun is reflected off it.)

Hallucinations

These are sensory experiences that cannot be verified by the direct experience of someone else who is present. In demented persons they are the result of brain damage that is part of the primary condition or the result of a superimposed delirium. Auditory or visual deficits in the patient can make these even worse since a double deficit—sensory and cognitive—is at work "scrambling the message." Most hallucinations in the demented appear to be visual and auditory, with a few olfactory in nature.[39]

It is best to counsel families that hallucinations should be evaluated by a physician, psychiatrist, neurologist, etc., to determine whether there is a physical basis for the hallucinations (delirium, a brain tumor, drug side effect, etc.). If no physical basis is found, psychoactive medication may be helpful in controlling or eliminating the hallucination. These are not always an effective therapy, and even if drugs should be successful, families/care-givers should be taught how to respond to the patient's hallucinations when they occur. Some suggestions include:

1. If the person is not upset by the hallucinations don't get aggressive about it. Calmly divert or distract the patient in a reassuring tone. Don't debate with the patient whether the hallucination is real. If it makes the person feel contented and doesn't interfere with the conduct of daily activity, let it be. ("That dog at the foot of your bed must make you feel less alone, Mrs. Black.") Reflect the feeling of companionship or security Mrs. Black requires without verifying the hallucination (Don't say: "Oh, it's a cute little dog").
2. If the hallucinations are frightening, or are prompting the patient to take action that could be dangerous in the long or short run, stay with the patient and calmly reassure him/her that you can help. Turn the lights on in a darkened room and stay with the patient (if the hallucination occurs at night) until he/she goes to sleep. If Mrs. Wilder says that she hears people trying to get into her room stay with her and tell her she'll feel calmer if someone is there. (Make sure nobody is really talking outside her door or outside under the window.)
3. DO NOT tell the patient that he/she is making it up, acting like a crazy person, driving you (the care-giver) out of your mind, or otherwise add fuel to the fires of anxiety. The patient is genuinely frightened by these phenomena, which are *very real*, and doesn't need to hear any more stressful news.
4. Finally, reassure families that these phenomena are not a sign of mental illness, or a signal that the patient will quickly deteriorate and become insane.

Delusions

Delusions are a disorder of thinking in which the person holds firmly onto false ideas that the rest of society does not believe. The demented person is most likely to have delusions in which people are trying to harm or control him/her or concerns about things being done to or happening in the body.[40] Delusions are difficult to argue about with a demented person because while they are based on a false premise, the cause-and-effect propositions that support the delusions are internally consistent but are incorrect as their "keystone" premise. A demented person's delusions are usually poorly systematized due to his/her impaired intelligence,[41] but are nevertheless unavailable for logical rebuttal. A recent study[42] found that thirty-one percent of all Alzheimer's disease-impaired subjects had delusions most of which involved the belief that people were stealing things from them. Nine percent believed that persons were plotting against them, to send them to jail, remove them from where they lived, or were trying to hurt them while helping them perform activities of daily living.

Delusions that involve unreal beliefs about the body ("I am rotting inside" or "My brain is gone") may indicate serious depressive affect and ideation arising from the person's feelings about lost physical integrity, and especially lost intellectual capacity. "My brain is gone" is a way of describing what he/she feels like in concrete terms. Some delusions are statements about self-esteem. "I'm rotting inside" is a concrete representation of the patient's depression-induced feelings "I am a rotten person." Other delusions, like the one in which a person says he/she is in danger because he/she is being controlled by outside "others,"—e.g., neighbors, or radio personalities—may represent a need for security and greater feelings of safety since he/she no longer feels adequate control of internal feelings. Still other delusions (e.g., grandiosity) are tied to the past history and experiences of the patient and as such represent an attempt to bolster the self-esteem that is caving in under the pressure of behavioral mistakes and maladaptive reactions caused by dementia.

Counselors should be prepared to help families/care-givers as they would in regard to the other related phenomena discussed above. As was stated before, families will do better when they understand that delusions are a signal that something is wrong with the patient's ability to process feelings and information. General intervention guidelines include:

1. The use of calm, reassuring tones and not responding with a challenge or debate about the delusion.
2. Checking with the physician to see whether an underlying physical difficulty has triggered the unusual thinking.
3. NEVER playing along in jest, use sarcasm, or hold the person up to ridicule. If the patient believes that he lives on a ship and is a sea captain, there is no reason to challenge this delusion unless and until his behavior becomes such that it is dangerous, or until his lack of cooperation poses a physical threat to himself or others (i.e., he yells, "Abandon ship we're sinking" in the

middle of lunch or refuses to follow directions because he insists that he's the captain and nobody gives him orders). In such an event psychiatric consultation is in order.
4. If the patient believes that he/she is the victim of a plot to harm him/her or is experiencing physical or mental difficulties because people are doing something to control his behavior or thinking, offer reassurance that you (the family member, caretaker, counselor) understand how upsetting this must be and will certainly tell them to stop. These delusions are often forgotten for a while and then recur, at which time the same intervention can be tried again. If the patient refuses to eat or take essential medicine (which is absolutely necessary), or will not come out of his/her room, a consultation with a psychiatrist can be of help.
5. Help the family to understand that accusations against them (such as that the spouse is having an affair, or that the caregiving son is accused by his patient-mother of cheating on her with that other woman [his wife]) are expressions of insecurity, low self-esteem and misinterpretations of reality. The spouse or child may need some counseling to deal with the feelings that can arise when such accusations are made, and support should be given in order to speak with the patient to try to correct the delusion ("I love you very much and you're the only woman/man I want" or "I am your son Jack, and that woman who lives here is my wife, Rebecca. You are my mother and I care about you very much).

Sundowning

Many families and professional care-givers find it very stressful when the patient, who might have been either manageable or a chore all day, gets worse each day in the late afternoon. As daylight fades and it grows dark, many demented patients can become more restless, confused, and anxious than they have been the rest of the day. The patient can become more demanding, less able to wait for things to be done or to happen, become more suspicious, disoriented, more easily upset and less able to pay attention and follow instructions. This is not a willful change of behavior, but is apparently a manifestation of the brain damage suffered by the patient.

The actual cause is not known, though it is possible that fatigue (many of us get tired toward five o'clock) or the effect of reduced illumination (making it difficult for the patient to pick up sensory cues) may play a role. The care-giver may have more to do (and therefore feels stressed and less able to pay attention to the patient) and may communicate impatience to the patient. It is also possible that a number of these factors are at work in such a way as to contribute to a cycle of increased agitation, feelings of greater anxiety about one's security and safety, impaired cognitive ability, greater caretaker stress, and physical discomfort and fatigue.

Families can be counseled to try to arrange their day's schedule so that more active, demanding things are done in the morning or early afternoon and more relaxing, passive activities take place later in the day and in the evening.[43,44] If the person is being cared for at home by a family care-giver, remind them that competition from other persons in need of their attention in the late afternoon (children returning home or the spouse returning from work) may generate rivalrous feelings for the care-giver in the patient who only understands that his/her needs must be met. Remember that fatigue brings a diminished ability to be patient and understanding in many of us, and the cognitively impaired are already less inclined to be patient and consider the feelings of others. In nursing homes, "sundowning" has long been thought to be a reaction to the day shift leaving at around 4–4:30 P.M., but the fact that sundowning occurs at home seems to suggest that there may be different reasons for it in each enviroment, or that factors common to both are the cause (diminishing light, increased fatigue, etc.). Some nursing homes have found that a brief rest or relaxation period before supper is helpful, as is a time when residents can say farewell to the day shift and welcome the evening shift.

Inability to Recognize People or Objects

Agnosia is the name given to the process by which the patient with dementia loses the ability to recognize a person or thing. This happens when the brain cannot match what the eyes see with its memories of once familiar stimulus patterns previously seen and stored. It can take the form of not knowing that a wastebasket is not a toilet, or that paper plates are not to be eaten, but it can also have a manifestation that is quite devastating to family members—failure to recognize who they are.

Many demented persons are unable to remember and thus recognize people and places that have long been familiar to them. There are instances when a patient will say that the person who claims to be a relative (spouse or sibling) is not that person, or is an impostor, or that the "real home" has been replaced with an identical substitute.[44]

People who are responded to in this way can feel very hurt and need reassurance that they are not being rejected by the patient, but are the victims of his/her inability to recognize and give meaning to stimuli that were once familiar. Insisting that the patient is mistaken will probably lead to greater behavioral difficulties for him/her, including angry outbursts or full-blown catastrophic reactions. Logic will not be understood, nor will pleas to the goodwill or mercy of the patient. The patient is unable to empathize with the unrecognized individual so cannot answer a question like "How do you think I feel when you don't know me?" It is best to calmly say to the patient, "You may not remember me, but I'm your daughter, Mary."

Clinging or Shadowing

A number of care-givers report that their demented relative or patient has the annoying pattern of following them wherever they go, even into the bathroom or when they go outside for a break. This can be most annoying since most people need to feel in control of their personal space, and require time to be alone to regroup and gather their thoughts. This is especially true for care-givers who are giving all day and look forward to a few minutes of solitude or a chance to "recharge their batteries." Being met by an angry or fretful dementia patient when you return from the bathroom or from a private moment in your room is quite stressful, and can provoke the care-giver to anger. One nurse reported that when she was in the nurses' station preparing medication one demented resident would come in and stand right next to her, only to be followed by a second who stood as close as she could to the first one, who was followed by a third, fourth, etc., until ten residents were all lined up with no space between them, anchored to this very trusted, security-providing nurse.

Clinging or shadowing is the patient's way of staying with a source of security and of finding reassurance that somebody who knows them and their needs is a constant in their ever-changing world. People with memory impairments cannot remember that when a person leaves their sight, he/she continues to exist even though he/she has temporarily vanished. They cannot preserve the image of you in their memory, so you do in fact disappear without a trace. Unlike the intact brain that can make correct estimates about the passage of time, the damaged brain can experience difficulties in estimating how much time has elapsed, so that five minutes seem like an hour. Time hangs especially heavy and passes most slowly when the cognitively impaired person is not doing anything. This is similar to the way young children experience the passage of time as a function of how much action they have engaged in. It is therefore a good idea to give the patient something to do as he/she accompanies the care-giver or awaits his/her return. Folding laundry, winding yarn around hangers, cardboard forms, into balls, etc., have worked well. Remember that the demented person is oriented toward his/her own needs, perceptions, comfort, and security, and will treat the care-giver in light of how these needs are met. The home-care provider may be able to arrange for relief if needed, so that privacy and respite can be built into his/her day and the patient will not be left feeling abandoned or unattended. Counseling can help family care-givers express feelings about the effects these behaviors have on them (i.e., make them angry, frustrated, want to scream) and be encouraged to obtain respite or relief help without feeling guilty. Such care-givers can benefit from counseling intervention that recognizes and supports their need for a life of their own and some enjoyment even though they are caring for a demented relative.

Depression, Apathy, and Withdrawal

Alzheimer's-disease patients may become depressed because they are somewhat aware that they are losing their mental abilities. They may feel like failures, like less of a person than they used to be, or feel sad but can't tell anyone why. Depression can exacerbate the memory impairment caused by Alzheimer's disease, thus making the patient feel even more out of control and like his/her mind is fading rapidly. It is not difficult to understand why an Alzheimer's patient would feel this way, or why he/she might choose to withdraw from life so as not to expose his/her disability to others and risk ridicule or lowered self-esteem. Patients who have been very demanding of themselves throughout life or perfectionistic may lose interest in doing anything when they have become even mildly impaired because their efforts will not be "good enough." Demented patients may become sad, tearful, dejected, and even express a wish to die. One demented patient repeatedly told her physician that if he wanted to help her he would kill her because she no longer wished to live.

Alzheimer's patients can develop a reaction that qualifies as a clinical depression, with appetite disturbances, weight loss, apathy, lack of enjoyment of formerly enjoyed activities, and guilt feelings. This may be due to a change in the neurochemistry of the brain, and may be treatable with drugs. Supportive counseling, activity, encouraging socialization, and the continued pursuit of retained or dormant interests and skills can do a great deal to help alleviate depression, withdrawal, and apathy in Alzheimer's patients. Telling them to get off their rear ends or to snap out of it, or attempting to cheer them up is usually counterproductive and leads to feelings of lowered self-worth since the patient feels that nobody really understands him/her. The patient may respond well to a gradual program of resocialization, first with one trusted friend or relative and later gradually increasing the number of visitors or persons doing the activity. Care-givers can promote and encourage any positive social behavior the person will engage in, no matter how simple it appears to be. It is the risk the patient feels able to take, and if successful, will be the basis for future success.

It is important that families understand that depression, apathy, and withdrawal are understandable reactions to becoming demented. While we can perhaps see ways to rationalize or cope with the problem, we can certainly sympathize with the patient's feelings of great loss and hopelessness when he/she becomes aware of being memory impaired. Families should be helped to appreciate the basis of these reactions, and to accept the fact that they are not vindictive responses to dementia designed by the patient to get back at the family.

Suicide

Upon learning of my interest in Alzheimer's disease, an old friend of mine whom I hadn't seen in years told me that his father had suffered from it. I remarked that I had seen his father's obituary in the newspaper, and I offered my condolences. My friend remarked that his father had died falling out of a window, and that he hoped it had been a suicide. If it had been, he said, it would have been his father's last rational act since he was unwilling to live as a demented person any longer. I was unable to ask how the rest of his family felt about this, but my old friend was clearly comforted by the possibility that his father had chosen how to die.

The demoralization, depression, and hopelessness that Alzheimer's patients can feel do not always lead to suicide, but the risk is obviously there. Impaired cognition may make planning a suicide difficult, but it is a good idea to reduce the opportunity and eliminate means by removing weapons, poisons, medications, car keys, power tools, razor blades, or other potential instruments of self-destruction. Dangerous windows and doors leading to busy thoroughfares should also be kept locked or secured. As my friend's remarks indicated, an impulse to act can have dire consequences.

Counselors may have to work with family members' feelings about issues of suicidal ideation, gestures, or actual successful attempts. Some families may react with anger at what they see as the patient's attempts to abandon or reject them by wishing to die, while others may secretly or openly feel relief or welcome the suicidal act as an indication of rationality and of the patient's having regained some control over life and death. It is important to review with the family their values, religious beliefs, and feelings about death in counseling about this issue. Care should be taken not to try to get the family to adopt the counselor's beliefs in an attempt to reduce or magnify any grief reactions or other emotional expression. If the patient makes an unsuccessful attempt at suicide, it may be appropriate to counsel him/her and help to give words to the patient's feelings.

Conclusion

The problem behaviors discussed in this chapter occur with countless variations in dementia patients, but are not always manifested by every one of them. There are also some kinds of problem behaviors that have not been discussed, and successful interventions devised by care-givers for some of these that likewise have not been mentioned here. It is important to remember that these problem behaviors are attempts by the patients to adapt to the environment as he/she interprets it, ways that bespeak an interpretation and a worldview that is at variance with our own. In essence, these behaviors seem to be the patient's attempt to "fit in" to a flow of behavior as best as he/she can understand it.

These difficulties are likely to produce discomfort in care-givers when they first occur, and may make the care-giver feel unsure about what will take place next. This feeling signals an imbalance in power, at odds with what is normally found in human relationships. Such behaviors may lead to feelings of anxiety, due to loss of control of the interaction, fear, and other similar responses to what the care-giver recognizes as a human interaction in which he/she does not know what to expect. This represents a skewing of the typical power distribution found in the (professional) care-giver-client (patient) relationship and in usual family interaction styles. When such internal expectations are violated by the odd or erratic behavior of another, responses by the observer designed to regain control of the interaction are likely to be provoked. Such reactions may include prohibiting or otherwise limiting the "deviant" behavior, using moral pressure ("You shouldn't steal other people's things; how would you like if they did that to you?"), attempts to prompt a more acceptable response ("You remember that you should wear clothes when you're out of your room, don't you Mrs. Smith?"), or similar interventions designed to restore a more comfortable "normal" balance of control within the interaction by eliciting more "normal" behavior. Professionals may be particularly uncomfortable when these behaviors occur suddenly and unpredictably because they are so used to being in control when interacting with clients. It is not unusual and certainly not unprofessional to experience fear, discomfort, wishes to escape, or a feeling of anxiety or tension when these problem behaviors are first witnessed. The care-giver—professional or family-care provider—ought to understand that this is a reasonable initial response that may require a decent interval of time and repeated exposures to such behaviors before more objective nonemotional responses take priority.

If these behaviors are properly understood by care-givers to be what they are—manifestations of disordered thought by often-frightened patients with damaged brains—a therapeutic response to them is more likely. Professional care-givers to the demented (nurse's aides, nurses, social workers, activity leaders, etc.) are frequently asked to contend with the worst of these behaviors in their service settings, and typically do so with aplomb. Emotional objectivity about the patient certainly helps, but understanding the bases of cognitive impairments appears to make the real difference. When asked if they get upset or angry by these behavioral problems, insightful care-givers usually reply that they can't get angry or upset because they understand that "when Harry hits me when I'm giving him a bath, I understand that he can't help it. I just say to myself, 'That's Harry!'"

Care-givers must often learn new ways to restore control when these behaviors occur, and recognize that the object of their intervention is to help the *patients* attain the ability to behave in a more controlled way. This may mean that the care-giver will have to accept a compromise with the patient about which alternative behavior can be evoked at a given moment to replace a particular problem behavior that has arisen because of the patient's cognitive impairment. Experience with dementia patients quickly teaches that some control (diversion or channeling) is better than none, and that one frequently faces situations where the patient will retain proportionally more control than the care-giver even though the acute behavioral problem has subsided due to appropriate intervention. Furthermore, struggles for power and control of interactions with demented persons are likely to be lost by care-givers/family members. All participants in the interaction may be left with a significant emotional residue that adds a negative, anxious, or fearful tone to future interactions, and that can result in poorer adaptation for the patient.

7

Assessing Service Needs, Finding Resources, and Making Referrals

It will be the job of many counselors to help patients and families identify needs, find resources in a particular community, accomplish referrals, and monitor the degree to which the patients' and families' needs are being met. Unless they are clinicians whose job it is to assess and intervene in the area of cognitive function per se, most counselors will tend to focus on the gamut of care needs that a particular Alzheimer's-disease patient must receive in order to achieve maximal adaptation to his/her environment.

A number of specific goals for care have recently been summarized.[1] Those pertaining to the current discussion include:

A. To preserve maximum independence of the patients.
B. To coordinate care provision efficiently across the full range of a continuum of care so that the best possible match is made between available services and the needs and preferences of the patient and family.
C. To reduce the severity of symptoms.
D. To preserve the dignity of the patient.
E. To maximize the use of abilities that remain and minimize the maladaptive effects of disabilities.
F. To treat medical problems that may exacerbate disabilities or cause pain or discomfort.
G. To promote family integrity and organization.

These goals set out broad guidelines for service by which counselors can determine the suitability and quality of care services they might choose to recommend. Counselors who have not had much prior exposure to the problems of Alzheimer's-disease patients and their families might experience some confusion about just what services ought to accomplish. Since Alzheimer's is a degenerative, presently incurable disorder, counselors will have to set aside any "cure" orientation they may normally utilize as a basis for thinking about the goals of their efforts.

Newcomers to the area of providing services to Alzheimer's-disease patients are often frustrated by the lack of a single, comprehensive service provider capable of meeting the diverse and changing needs of these patients. Families and other service providers are frustrated as well by the need to develop an aggregation of services for each patient, and to coordinate this "package" lest it fall down in a domino-like effect when one service is absent or unreliable, or becomes ineffective due to a change in the patient's condition.

In a recent survey,[2] care-givers to the demented were asked to assess the importance of various services regardless of cost or availability. The ten services they rated as most essential were:

A. A paid companion to provide in-home respite for care-givers a few hours per week.
B. Assistance in finding patient-care resources.
C. Assistance in applying for government programs (e.g., Medicare, Medicaid, disability insurance, and income support programs).
D. A paid companion for overnight respite so that care-givers can leave the house for one or more days.
E. Home care, such as assisting the patient with dressing or feeding.
F. Support groups.
G. Special nursing-home programs exclusively for dementia patients.
H. Short-term respite in health-care institutions (acute and long-term care)
I. Adult day-care centers.
J. Visiting nurses' service in the home.

Silverstein and Hyde[3] report that respite, homemaker, adult day-care, home-health aide and nursing-home information were the five services most requested by care-givers to Alzheimer's patients. Care-givers seem to be feeling that they can carry the major burdens of care giving with the aid of some specific and limited assistance in clearly defined areas of need. Counselors might take this data into account when talking with families about their need for care services. The counselor can ask the care-giver to rate those services he/she feels are most required for the immediate future, and those that might be required long range. The nine-step counseling model discussed in this book is a useful method to apply to such a task, particularly steps 3–8, which help a client (caretaker) become specific about needs in the midst of an often-chaotic situation.

For those new to the myriad of resources an Alzheimer's-disease patient and his/her family might possibly need, a look at appendix B will help them to become familiar with the care services Alzheimer's-disease and other dementia patients and their families might require. It lists care services which would be potentially beneficial but which may not be universally available.

Making a Referral

For most of the readers of this book, a referral to one or a number of additional services will be an inevitable component of counseling. The wide range of ever-changing needs and the real limitations as to what any one service provider can achieve in meeting the multifold care requirements of an Alzheimer's patient dictate that referral and linkage to other service providers will be necessary. Successful referrals require:

1. Accurate assessment of needs.
2. Good communication of the assessment results to the patient, if possible, and to the care-giver.
3. Cooperation by the patient.
4. Cooperation by the care-giver.
5. Availability of a service resource(s) to meet the service need.

The aim of the referral should be clearly in mind when it is made, and can be formulated so as to specify what important clinical information might be derived or, alternatively, what specific clinical need will be met. (For example, "I am referring Mr. Jones to you to see whether he has any physical illness which might be causing some confusion" or "Could Mr. Jones use some therapy to help him maintain ambulation?") Knowing the aim of your referral will also help "sell" the referral to skeptical professionals who may not be sure about what help they can be with regard to an Alzheimer's patient.

Assessment

While memory loss, language ability, or spatial reasoning can be measured in demented individuals, it is unclear how a given level of these or other capacities as reflected in standardized tests contributes to an understanding of a patient's level of day to day adaptation.[4,5,6,7] Appraisal of the patient's ability to do the practical self-care activities is a more useful contribution to the family/care-giver than is a battery of tests that measures cognitive abilities. The counselor should bear this in mind, and with the family/care-giver, develop an inventory of those activities of daily living with which the patient needs help (eating, dressing, communication, etc.) Specific hints about how to help will make this appraisal more meaningful and help the patient's actual adaptation to the environment.

Cognitive capacity of the patient contributes to but does not determine the entire nature of caregiver burden. The care-giver actually has three types of burdens and all should be evaluated. Besides the physical caregiving such as bathing, dressing, supervising, etc., there are the emotional burdens and cognitive burdens the care-giver must contend with. The former include coping with the personal feelings the caretaker has regarding his/her loss of freedom and autonomy, the deterioration and loss of a loved one, and the resentment, sadness, and anger that accompany such an experience and endless demands on his/her time. The cognitive tasks of the caretaker involve the additional anticipatory and interpretive thinking the care-giver must do in order to "understand" the behavior of the patient. This work involves decoding communication from a person with impaired language, guessing what the patient will do next or what the impact of a certain word, event, or decision might be on the patient, and altering usual ways of doing things and thinking about day-to-day life that were developed and internalized before the person became a care-giver. Each dementia victim and her/his care-giver(s) will present the counselor with a unique amalgam of behavioral difficulties and care burdens that require assessment and intervention on an individual basis.[8]

Communicating the Results

Care-givers, especially family members, are prone to ask clinicians: "What stage is she in?" or "How long before she won't recognize me?" or "When will I know that he/she needs to be in a nursing home?" Functional assessments available today do not have the ability to designate with total accuracy a stage of dementia, nor can they predict the rate of future cognitive deterioration. There are also no instruments available to determine readiness for institutionalization, since this is a function of whether care needs can be met by family and/or community-based care-givers and it is not simply a matter of how severely impaired the patient is.

The results of the functional assessments are useful primarily as indicators of current functions and to catalogue abilities and disabilities in concrete ways so that the goals of intervention are clearer than if a care-giver were to be told how many words the patient could not remember. Communicating the results of the assessment(s) to the care-giver (usually the family) is primarily an opportunity to provide a *systematic*, organized picture of what he/she will be called upon to do for the patient, and to ascertain his/her willingness and ability to do what is required. Counseling can be an important method by which the care-giver(s):

1. Learns to accept and cope with feelings about the reality of the patient's abilities and disabilities.
2. Examines honestly and in an objective, unbiased atmosphere (unlike many family discussions on the subject) whether he/she feels that care-giving can be continued and if so, to what extent and in which area of disability.
3. Can learn to express and cope with feelings about working as part of a team for the future care of their relative.
4. Is provided with objective, behavioral data rather than observations colored by the emotional needs of the observer on which to base care-planning projections.
5. Can participate in developing a comprehensive, integrated plan of care that can be utilized with the assessment as a basis for service planning.
6. Can interact with the counselor to determine whether individual care-givers might profitably be referred for counseling or informational assistance to help contend with the emotional and cognitive burdens of care.

Eliciting Patient Cooperation

Ultimately it is the patient who has to agree to attend or cooperate with a care resource. Care-givers frequently get encouraged when a resource is found that appears to meet the patient's and their needs, only to become frustrated when the patient resists going or attends and announces that he/she will "never go back to that place." In the same vein, families can become very annoyed when their patient or relative refuses to allow in-home services to be performed, or discharges the paid care-giver.

The patient's cooperation is not simply a function of how cognitively impaired he/she is. Some patients become more accepting of help when their dementia worsens. That is, at mild levels of impairment they tend to resist assistance and deny any problems, but cease resisting and cooperate when they are moderately or severely demented. Other patients are cooperative while they still maintain enough cognitive and linguistic abilities to respond to explanations, coaxing, or negotiation, and become resistant or uncooperative when they are more impaired and unable to understand what is being done or what is expected of them.

It is usually a good idea to explain to the patient what is to happen and elicit his/her cooperation and assent to attend a day-treatment center or to go to the doctor. Sometimes counselors or care-givers can get anxious about whether the client will agree to go along with the plan and beat around the bush while using complicated sentences that disguise their real message. Besides communicating any fears or anxiety they have, counselors or care-givers who communicate this way flood the patients with messages that are difficult to comprehend and therefore can result in frustration, anger, and low self-esteem ("Boy, am I really losing my mind! I can't understand what I'm being told but he [the speaker] seems to think I should understand him.")

Patients will have questions about what they are being told, and may or may not be able to formulate them. They may worry about whether anyone will know who they are (remember, *THEY* can't remember who most other people are), or if someone at home will remember to get them to bring them home at the end of the day. Concerns may also exist about what will happen to them while they are there, such as if they'll get fed or taken to the bathroom. Many of these and other concerns may not be articulated due to their being unconscious or because the patient cannot put these worries into words, and may be manifested as anxiety, preoccupation, clinging dissatisfaction, somatic complaints, or negativism. If these behaviors are seen and some emotional conflict about a referral to a community-based service is suspected, it can be helpful to the client if he/she is reminded where it is that he/she is going, how long he/she will stay, and what the purpose of the excursion is to be. If the care-giver will be staying with the client—a useful transitional and adjustment strategy in many cases—that should be told to the client as well.

The personality of the patient is an important variable in eliciting cooperation. Temperament or personality has been found to remain stable over the life span[9] and it constitutes a major dimension in determining the outcome of a patient's reaction to a new situation. Just as there are wide variations in behavioral manifestations of dementia among patients, so too are there considerable individual differences in personality that constitute the substrate of the patient's reactions to new or unexpected experiences. Though memory and other aspects of cognition may deteriorate and impair the patient's social skills, his/her reaction to social situations are likely to be affected in some manner by a combination of intrinsic, relatively stable lifelong tendencies in such situations, as well as by the patient's appraisal (a cognitive task) or awareness of his/her skills and competency in that setting. This appraisal may be on target or not depending upon whether the patient can accurately determine which of his/her current social skills are congruent or incongruent with the demands of the social situation. An accurate appraisal yields "appropriate behavior," while an inaccurate one leads to behavior usually termed dysfunctional, "socially inappropriate" or worse, "infantile" and "regressed." But the patient's inclination based on intrinsic emotional reactions will play a large role in determining how comfortable an experience will be.

If, for example, the person is gregarious and has lived a life built around the satisfaction of this tendency, group activities might be a positive setting in which the person can utilize residual social and cognitive skills. A more introverted person or a person who prefers solitude may find this an anxiety-producing setting, in which his/her remaining social and cognitive capacities are subordinated to responding to the anxiety and discomfort that arise. Some people can be described as "slow to warm up."[10] These individuals take a little time to adjust at their own rate and if encouraged to do so, will likely adapt.

Taking the personality of the patient into account is also a useful thing to do when informing the patients of an upcoming referral. (A good personal history of the patient obtained during the appraisal can be very helpful.) If the person is a worrier who constantly ruminates about things, telling him/her in advance may not be a good idea. Rather, it may be advisable for the care-giver to discuss the new arrangement as part of the day's events prior to beginning preparations for leaving. Individuals who like to exercise their choices about things might be approached as follows:

> COUNSELOR: There is a group of people like yourself who meet for lunch every day. They are friendly people, like yourself, and are looking for new friends all the time. I think if you went you could have a great time. Would you like to go?

Notice that memory problems, old people, respite for the caregiver (a useful side benefit of such a referral) or any "therapeutic" benefit to be gained from attending were not mentioned. Demented people may worry about acceptance, looking "stupid" if they need help with their memory (if they are aware of their diminishing social and linguistic skills), and whether it will be all right with the caregiver (i.e., will the care-giver be unhappy or worry if they attend). They may wonder whether they can they get the care-giver to approve and thereby validate the proposed experience as being acceptable or good for the client. Client cooperation with in-home services is influenced by the same variables. Persons with strong antidependency feelings, or who are fearful of loss of control over their environment may reject in-home help. Persons who are more dependent may be more likely to accept it better.

Persons with dementia develop a sense of trust or mistrust in their care-giver such that an enthusiastic invitation to do something (e.g., go to a nutrition program) is acceptable because of the faith the patient has in the judgment of the care-giver. Care-givers often speak about behavioral contagion among Alzheimer's and other dementia patients, where if one person gets upset, others around him/her do so as well. This phenomenon works with positive emotions as well. The most skilled and effective care-givers succeed because they convey an attitude of warmth, acceptance, and enthusiasum for what they do, and because they truly care about the people they care for. This attitude comes through in their interactions with their patients/clients and their relatives, and promotes security and risk taking when the care-giver suggests that something is positive or might be fun. Consider the effect of saying enthusiastically to a person with dementia: "They're having lunch down at the church. What do you say about you and I going and having some fun?" versus the detached care-giver who deadpans: "It's time for you to go to the lunch program now." Enthusiasm and optimism can be contagious, and are helpful motivators for demented people. The emotions conveyed must be genuine, however, or the process will fail miserably. Demented persons are superb at distinguishing affective (emotional) messages in speech, and in fact can discern emotional cues in communication even when they are unable to produce intelligible speech and are significantly intellectually impaired.[11]

Family care-givers often feel great conflict about turning over some or all of the patient's care to "strangers," so this transition can be a stressful time. This conflict and stress, and the guilt, sadness, anger, and other feelings that may occur make it harder for family care-givers to communicate with the patient about the need for the service. Instead, they fear exposing their guilt and ambivalence. Modeling how to discuss a referral is therefore stress reducing, and imparts to the referral an air of legitimacy because it is presented in a positive, nondisguised way.

Cooperation by the Care-giver

The above-mentioned feelings, especially ambivalence, can lead a family care-giver to appear to be resistant and uncooperative. The process of recognizing that the care-giver cannot do it all can provoke a crisis for that family member. As was discussed in the chapter on the family, there are many family dynamics and "contracts" that make care giving to an angry parent or sibling an opportunity for redemption, martyrdom, an object lesson, or preferably, the continuation of a caring, positive relationship. So while a family care-giver may recognize his/her own stress and the patient's need for service, feelings may get in the way of following through on what the care-giver knows to be best for everyone.

That is not to say that all objections or disagreements by caretakers about referral are a result of emotional factors. There may be legitimate concern about any referral, and the counselor should take this seriously. All of the questions, objections or reservations about referral deserve a fair, objective hearing by the counselor. Even though the professional has worked very hard to assess a patient's needs and find appropriate services, the care-giver usually knows the patient and the practical realities of his/her life situation best and should be treated as an equal team member with unique insight and information to contribute.

If the counselor suspects resistance on the part of the care-giver for any particular reason, he/she can proceed to discuss the care-giver's feelings about the referral. Is the need for service, the agency, or the provider a problem? The counselor may choose to explore whether the feelings of the care-giver emanate from his/her own emotional milieu (e.g., family pressures not to surrender any aspects of care, overattachment to the parent, denial of the disorder, etc.) or from feelings about objective aspects of the referral itself (e.g., distance from home, other participants the patient is liable to find at a service site, or dissatisfaction with the provider based on a previous contact). In either case, a compromise can often be negotiated in which the care-giver agrees to implement certain acceptable components of the service plan while others remain under discussion in counseling.

Service Availability and Meeting Service Needs

The service need of any patient with Alzheimer's or other dementia is composed of two primary factors. The first is the area of deficit and function where intervention is necessary, e.g., recreational or occupational therapy, assistance with activities of daily living, etc. The second is the requirement that the service provider and/or service setting be appropriate and acceptable to the patient and his/her caretakers. But the service most suitable to providing assistance in a given area of need must first and foremost be available on a regular, reliable basis. Many communities are currently recognizing the gulf that lies between token availability and the substantial, actual presence of a particular service component. The counselor making a referral should determine whether a service provider has the resources in personnel, available program slots for clients, geographic catchment area, transportation if necessary, daily availability, etc., to meet a particular client's needs. Other service providers, professionals in the local community, and former or present clients are good sources of feedback about a service provider's performance record.

This issue of reliability and availability is so very important for the counselor to determine because the credibility of the counselor as a referral source, the credibility of the referred-to agency, and the quality of life for the patient and his/her caretaker are at stake when any referral is made. Alzheimer's patients and their care-giver's frequently report intense frustration with referrals that prove to be illusory when it turns out that the agency or provider to whom they have been referred cannot deliver the service due to high staff turnover, no vacancies in a program, inadequate ability to meet the actual need of the patient on a regular basis, etc. In sum, the counselor making a referral has a responsibility to make such referrals based on current information about the performance record of the prospective provider and not just on the basis of its publicity or claims. Remember that once the family or other care-giver has gone through the process of "letting go" of their patient and has agreed to engage other services, they can respond with great anger and frustration to the additional stress of a referral that has fallen through or has not been reliable, appropriate or competent. Such circumstances can make them feel more guilt than they did before they accepted help, because they may feel responsible for the existence of these additional unhappy circumstances for the patient and themselves.

A prospective service provider for Alzheimer's disease and related-disorder sufferers should at minimum provide evidence of having expertise in helping this population, either by the presence of successfully adapted dementia clients in their service population group or by other indices, such as the presence of workers trained by qualified authorities in Alzheimer's care. Though it is not necessary that the entire caseload of the provider agency be comprised of Alzheimer's disease or other dementia patients (an integrated setting or service caseload can be a positive indicator about a provider), the provider should be able to give some evidence that it is aware of the special-care need these patients have and knows how to respond to them. Any evidence of bias against such patients or ignorance of what causes their adaptional and behavioral difficulties (such as calling them "just senile" or tendencies toward infantilization, e.g., "We love them all to death, they're all just like our children") should arouse the counselor's suspicion and stimulate further investigations about their expertise.

A service provider qualified to care for demented clients should also give some evidence of the fact that he/she understands that persons with Alzheimer's and related disorders find it difficult to adjust to new settings and new people. When the patient fails to do so it is not necessarily that he/she is being obstinant, negativistic, or selfish, but perhaps because his/her cognitive impairments make it difficult for him/her to adapt. An indication by the provider that he/she expects the demented person to do the adapting to an inflexible structure that will not respond to individual client needs and capacities is a warning that the patient may have trouble "fitting in."

Finally, a service provider or resource should be willing to cooperate with the referral source who is continuing ongoing treatment of the patient or family, with the family itself, and with other providers. Remember that the typical service package utilized by an Alzheimer's-disease or other demented patient is likely to be a series of services linked by a care-giver or other manager of care. This requires that the individual service providers be willing to work toward the same goals, without fighting over who has the best interest of the patient at heart or to whom the patient "truly belongs." Doing so harms the patient. Such power struggles take the vulnerable patient and utilize him/her as a conduit of messages about how one provider feels about the other, much as behaviorally disturbed children can be "triangulated" when communication between parents becomes dysfunctional.[12]

A good service provider will also be aware of the impact Alzheimer's and related diseases have on families, especially when family members are care-givers. It will recognize that the family/care-giver is also a service recipient and encourage communication between the family and the service provider(s). It does not help the patient if family members are treated as villains instead of as victims, no matter how difficult or uncooperative they may become.

8

Counseling and Residential Long-term Care Placement of the Alzheimer's Victim

The great physical, emotional, and financial burdens of caring for a demented relative at home are more easily borne by some families than is the decision to institutionalize the patient. The length of time a family can continue to provide such care is influenced by the amount of "care-giver burden" it feels it can assume and the point at which each individual family feels it can no longer sustain home care because the burden has become too great.[1] It is not clear, however, why some families continue to provide care as their burden intensifies and puts care-givers at risk, while others are willing to turn the care of their patients over to professional care-givers. Primary factors leading to institutionalization include problems of coping with the disturbed behavior of the patient, lack of adequate outside help and respite, and financial difficulties eventuating from the conduct of care.[2] A recent study by Colerick and George[3] found that severity of symptoms or level of cognitive disability are not sufficient to explain why a decision to seek nursing-home placement is made at a given time. Their data suggest that the structure and characteristics of the care-giver support system are instead better predictors of institutional placement. It is noteworthy that they also found that relinquishing the care of the demented relative does not necessarily seem to relieve care-giving burden as one would expect it to. Clinical experience with care-giving families suggests that one of the major sources of continued stress is the emotional aftermath following placement, particularly feelings of guilt.

As community-based services grow in response to the increased awareness our society has developed about the needs of Alzheimer's-disease victims, placement in a long-term care facility can be forestalled, and in many instances, prevented. While long-term care used to be synonymous with institutional placement, there are a growing number of community-based long-term care services that have developed around the country that permit prolonged maintenance of dementia patients in the home. Though services are not abundantly available and cannot therefore meet the totality of needs that the demented population in any community presents, a positive beginning is under way.[4,5] There are also generally not enough nursing-home beds available in most communities, and many facilities have made it a practice to exclude demented applicants because of reimbursement constraints, the perceived or actual disruptive effect of demented persons on the nondemented residents and other reasons.[6]

A recent comprehensive report on programs and services for persons with dementia[7] reports the following residential care alternatives:

1. SHORT-TERM RESIDENTIAL CARE—also called respite-residential care. Provides the patient with a stay of a few days or weeks, usually in a long-term care facility. This service is not widely available, and has some noticeable drawbacks, including patients' difficulties adjusting to transfer, reluctance of families to resume care of the patient at the end of the agreed-upon respite period, and, if respite is given in an acute-care setting, great expense.
2. FOSTER HOMES, DOMICILIARY CARE, BOARDING HOMES—these residential care facilities vary in size, licensing requirements, and state regulation of their care. There are a small number of exemplary residences in this category, but they nevertheless demonstrate that Alzheimer's and related disorder patients can be cared for and thrive outside of medical model long-term residential care. This is particularly true for mildly to moderately impaired persons.[8]
3. HOSPICE—these assist demented patients near the end of life by providing psychosocial, pastoral, and medical care to the patient and family members. Since the terminal phase of dementia can last for years, many families seek to arrange appropriate but not aggressive medical care for the patient who is nearing the end of life.[9] Families may be able to benefit from such services available in their communities and may be able to be assisted by counseling to decide upon placement and cope with the emotional reactions they have as a result of it.

Special Care for Dementia in Nursing Homes

A number of resources are available to assist with this phase of counseling. A book such as *Choosing a Nursing Home* by Richards et al (University of Washington Press, 1985) and *You and Your Aging Parent* by B. Silverstone and H. Hyman (Consumers Union, 1982) are two of the more helpful books currently available.

Medical model nursing homes as they have traditionally been organized have not been terribly well suited to caring for Alzheimer's patients.[10] As a result, many have begun to develop special-care units and programs to provide specialized care for the demented. Whether they are the outcome of the belief that special care will benefit both the demented and nondemented residents together, or of astute marketing strategies that recognize the demographics of aging and dementia,[11] they are proliferating everywhere. In the absence of any standards as to what specialized dementia care ought to be if it is to be "special," families may be vulnerable to the hyperbolic, hard-sell public-relations strategies of some facilities. These providers make promises in a general way so that enough of what families wish for and need to hear to reduce their fears during the time they are considering placement is communicated. Families are further handicapped when there is pressure to place the patient if he/she is in an acute-care setting. The public's lack of sophistication as to what can be done for dementia patients often contributes to a placement decision justified in large part by a facility's claim to have an "Alzheimer's Unit" that exists in name only.

Families often require advice and counsel when the time comes to consider placement of their demented relative. Counselors can be of significant assistance if they know some of the specific features that characterize specialized care for the demented in long-term care facilities. The debate about the benefit of specialized care units is a vigorous one,[12,13,14,15,16] and suggests that special care for dementia victims—whether on a "special unit" or not—can positively influence quality of life.

Until more data are available, families will have to become comfortable with personally evaluating a special-care program in a long-term care facility and drawing a conclusion as to whether their relative will be well cared for in that particular environment. Families will face the issue of an institution's practice of caring for dementia patients on a segregated unit versus whether they live among nondemented residents. This distinction is hotly debated and by itself says very little about the QUALITY of care residents receive in either setting. Families should be advised to look for the presence of a special program designed to meet the cognitive, emotional, and physical needs of dementia patients. A special unit does not necessarily offer specialized care, and it may in fact simply signify the segregation of demented persons to avoid bothering other, intact residents, and the staff. Segregation by itself is not a means by which to deliver special care; it may in fact constitute a way to deliver substandard treatment out of anyone's sight.

To create opportunities for the residents of a special-care unit for Alzheimer's and other dementias to flourish, the unit should be oriented toward creating conditions where the demented person can utilize his/her competencies and not be at risk due to dysfunction. Specialized care should be philosophically rooted in the goal of increasing the likelihood of a match between the person's abilities and what the environment encourages and permits him/her to do in order to flourish. Care should be individualized, innovative, and evolving. If this is the case, a resident in a special-care program—whether based on a homogeneous placement model (special-care unit) or a heterogeneous, integrated living model—will be able to enjoy feelings of safety, competency, satisfaction, self-esteem, and joy.

Families or other care-givers considering placement on a special-care unit for Alzheimer's and related disorders should evaluate whether the program meets the following criteria:[17,18]

1. Provides a program of stimulation that reduces illness and promotes prosocial, adaptive behaviors used in everyday life, thus eliminating emotional stress and excess disability brought about by withdrawal of interest from an impoverished environment;
2. Provides an environment that is appropriately modified to enhance chances at successful adaptation and reduce the chances of physical injury;
3. Encourages social interaction with peers, staff, visitors, and volunteers utilizing role-valorizing[19] social settings, and maximally safe autonomy;
4. Prevents excess disability due to physical, social, or psychological causes;

5. Provides staff who are trained, supervised, and supported so that they encourage resident autonomy and in so doing, become empowered and reinforce their own sense of autonomy and pride;
6. Provides staff members who meet resident's dependency needs in a dignified way without infantalization or the inducement of excess disability through creating overdependency, and who allow the resident to exercise remaining autonomous functions;
7. Creates an environment that is dignified, personalized, predictable, has informational redundancy to help with orientation, and supports a dignified self-image for the residents;
8. Manages wandering, agitation, unpredictable behavior, abusive language, etc., in policy, procedure, and care-planning contexts as signs of the person's cognitive disorder (not simply by labeling it as "acting out," "infantile," "regressed behavior," or other misapplied jargon) and has staff intervene by prevention or adaptation-facilitating responses;
9. Uses as few physical restraints and psychoactive drugs as possible, and utilizes these to benefit the resident's well-being rather than as a response to staff or family stress (counseling is the treatment of choice for the latter two groups when they become upset with the demented person's behavior);
10. Tends to the emotional and informational needs of the families, staff, and nondemented residents through appropriate means (e.g., support groups, in-service training, stress-reduction training, resident meetings, etc.);
11. Assesses a resident's problem behaviors in an objective, nonjudgmental way so as to discover the triggers, if any, in staff interaction, inappropriate programming, physical-medical problems, etc.;
12. Provides or requires a preadmission evaluation for dementia for diagnostic, care planning and reevaluation purposes to rule out diagnoses of dementia rendered without adequate exploration as to etiology and to evaluate the resident's response to and suitability for different care options;
13. Uses an approach that mixes structure, autonomy, flexibility, and creativity to promote the suitability and therapeutic impact of the program for each individual resident; and

14. Recognizes that everything need not be called "therapy" in order to establish its validity as an experience that is worthwhile for demented people, and that to do so reinforces the "sick role" of the resident and the "wellness" of the staff.[20]

The Dilemmas of Placement in Long-term Care

Family members differ widely in how well they accept the need for long-term care placement of their demented relative and may show a wide range of emotional reactions once placement has occurred. Counselors can be better prepared to assist family members if they keep in mind that the usually negative reactions relatives have to institutional placement in general can be intensified when a relative with Alzheimer's disease or similar dementia requires nursing-home care. Perhaps because the patient looks healthy or is so unable to assert his/her own needs and is so dependent, or because turning the care of a demented relative over to strangers is feared to be the breach of a trust, relatives may have a uniquely difficult time when placement occurs.

Positive coping to placing a relative in a nursing home involves initial acceptance, reality and awareness of loss, pulling back, grieving the loss, working through, establishing a healthy emotional distance, and acceptance. Negative coping is described as being characterized by guilt and/or anger at the patient or the self, denial of real issues, overinvolvement or flight, projection of anger onto staff, blaming the staff and harboring unrealistic expectations of staff and patient, unresolved guilt with an inability to separate, and dysfunction.[21] This description is helpful as an orientation schema for the counselor's thinking, but it has not yet been empirically validated as a universal description of what actually occurs.

Case Illustration: The Clayborns

Mr. Clayborn, seventy-eight years old, had been taken to the emergency room of the local hospital after he became agitated, verbally abusive, and struck his wife as she tried to stop him from leaving the house in his pajamas and bathrobe at 2:00 A.M. He was evaluated by a psychiatrist and psychologist, who suspected that he had probable mild to moderate progressive Alzheimer's-type dementia. It appeared that he also had an acute dementia secondary to the antipsychotic drug he had been given by his internist a few days before to control his agitation and restlessness. He was also suffering the dementing effects of a medication he was being given by his cardiologist. Consultations with these physicians achieved an agreement to alter his drug regime to see whether this would improve his cognition. The psychiatrist and psychologist also met with Mr. Clayborn's wife, an overwhelmed seventy-four-year-old retired nurse who appeared depressed and agitated, and their niece who lived some three hours away. She was their only relative and was clearly torn between wanting to help her uncle and aunt by assisting with his care after he was discharged, and the need to continue to meet her own family obligations.

Mrs. Clayborn expressed feelings of great anxiety about the future since she was not sure that she could care for her husband without help but did not want to place him in a nursing home. "The social worker says I should, that I can't take care of him. I can't do that to him. We've been married fifty-two years, and all we have is each other. He'll never forgive me if he goes into a home. No, I just couldn't do that to him! But where will I get the help I need to care for him? I can take care of him most of the time, but I'll need help a few hours a day. Maybe someone could live in. We have a third story on our home that could be a nice apartment. This way I'd sleep at night. You know I haven't had a full night's sleep in three years since he started with his memory problems."

When Mrs. Clayborn's response to placement and her interest in exploring an assessment and search for community-based services was discussed with the discharge planner, she replied, "She can't take care of him at home! She wants him in a nursing home. She told me that. She said she couldn't care for him alone. Besides, she can't manage him in spite of what she might say to you. I know what's best for her." Mrs. Clayborn's ambivalence and confusion were understandable reactions to her crisis, and were discussed as such with the discharge planner. She was under tremendous pressure to expedite Mr. Clayborn's transfer out of the hospital because his approved length of stay had run out, and the Clayborns were facing the prospect of having to pay the bill for the time spent in the hospital in excess of third-party insurer policies.

The facts indicated that Mrs. Clayborn was probably not truly able to care for her husband at home without extensive assistance by a home-health and homemaker agency, medical services, psychiatric follow-up and help with behavioral management of his wandering and outbursts of anger, but Mrs. Clayborn had to reach this conclusion on her own if it was going to be achieved without debilitating amounts of guilt and ambivalence. To this end, she agreed to have two counseling sessions with the psychologist in the next five days while her husband's application process for a nursing home was begun and he remained hospitalized. She was told that he did not have to go if she decided against it, but that if she felt it was a good idea that he go to a nursing home the process of requesting admission would be under way. The counseling allowed her to make her own decision in the face of the objective realities she was able to see when the pressure on her to comply with the discharge planner's opinion was eased. When her feelings about abandonment, guilt, and "broken contract" with her husband were explored, she decided for herself that in spite of these feelings, they would both be at risk if he came home. Her guilt, she said, would be less, knowing that she made the best decision she could under the circumstances.

Counseling for Mrs. Clayborn involved helping her recognize her strong commitment to her husband, her grief and sadness at his gradual departure from her life as spouse, companion, dominant person in the marriage, and her fears about her future without him. Her professional self-image required her to be able to take care of anyone (she had worked in a psychiatric hospital for a number of years) and so her self-esteem needed buttressing with regard to the differing realities of what she could do as a young nurse and what was possible at the age of seventy-four. This got her to look at her feelings about her own aging. When Mrs. Clayborn was able to express her own desires in counseling rather than to respond to what she thought others wanted her to say (and thereby gain approval and acceptance by pleasing them), she said that she couldn't take care of her husband alone, and was reluctant to rely on outside help that could prove to be unreliable, dishonest, or inadequate (not altogether untrue fears). She said she knew she was "supposed" to feel otherwise, but that that was her honest feeling. One month after placement she returned for another counseling session and asked for reassurance that she had done the right thing. Her predicament was reviewed, her feelings rearticulated, and she and the counselor agreed that she had done the best that she could have done at that time. When Mrs. Clayborn was allowed to determine what was in her own best interest, her decision was much more reassuring and comforting than it was when she was told what to do by someone else even though the outcome was the same. It is noteworthy that Mr. Clayborn was not placed in a special-care program for dementia, nor is he currently receiving any services designed to support his highest level of cognitive and psychosocial adaptation. Yet Mrs. Clayborn is satisfied that for the present time they are better off than if he were living at home.

Case Illustration: Mr. Rasmussen

Mr. Rasmussen began to experience subtle changes in memory when he was sixty-seven years old. A widower who had raised his seven children alone since his wife had died when their oldest was nine, he had begun to lose weight. He would forget what to buy at the grocery store and thus didn't eat much. His son lived nearby and began to look in on his father each week to prepare his grocery list and to take his father shopping. During the next three years Mr. Rasmussen's memory gradually became worse until he couldn't prepare meals, drive the car without getting lost, or remember the names of his grandchildren. His adult children decided that he was in danger if he lived alone, but that it was not feasible for him to live with any of them. Instead they sought placement at a long-term care facility that had a highly regarded program for persons with dementia. They hoped that he would be happier and function better for a longer period of time if he were in a specialized environment better suited to his needs and capabilities.

Though the family was satisfied with the program, some of the children were not without some sadness about their father's condition and the fact that he ended up in a long-term care facility. Some valid concerns they had about his treatment brought them to a counselor to discern how best to go about airing their complaints. The counselor was able to determine that Mr. Rasmussen's children actually had two issues or problems that needed attention. The first was their concern that their father's care was not being carried out in a manner consistent with who he was as a person and what his lifelong preferences were. A very private, religious man, he refused to be showered in the facility by a female staff member. His sense of modesty and his belief that only a man's wife should see him unclothed led him to become uncooperative when shower time came. The family felt that the staff at the facility did not know this about him since he could no longer express himself well verbally, and they were looking for a way to relate these facts about their father to the staff. They were angry and upset that nobody at the facility understood this, and that nobody had asked about his sense of modesty or bathing preferences before he was admitted. Their second issue, and the one about which they felt more anger and sadness, was their reaction to the fact that he had been institutionalized after he had raised all of them. Now, when he needed them, they couldn't take care of him. At this point one of the younger children expressed profound feelings of sadness about her mother's death, and said that she had never completely mourned that loss. She was discouraged from expressing her grief or from asking questions about her mother as she was growing up. When she began grieving the loss of her father, a process that family members of demented people often begin to do while the patients are still alive but dissolving as people,[22] unresolved grief about her mother reappeared and led her and some of her siblings to reconnect with their old feelings of sadness, anger, and sense of helplessness.

Counseling with this family was devoted to the four problems that had come up: The difficulty with the care plan and how to work with the facility to achieve a satisfactory solution for Mr. Rasmussen's bathing; the feelings of grief that some of the children were expressing about the change in their father and the process of losing him gradually as his cognition worsened; the related issue of their guilt about not being able to care for him and "repay the debt" they felt for the devotion and love he showed when he raised them single-handedly; and the younger child's unresolved grief about her mother's death and her feelings about how this event was dealt with by the family. This latter issue prompted her to reestablish contact with her former psychotherapist to work on this source of conflict. When these issues were separated and handled as four interrelated problems with different goals, alternatives for action, and possible conclusions and outcomes, the family was able to approach the facility with less anger, but with no less insistence, that their father's care arrangements be modified to respect his personal needs. In Mr. Rasmussen's case, a real care issue was the trigger for deep feelings to emerge that transcended the one problem and led to an exploration of feelings about his dementia, placement, and other losses the family had suffered.

Things to remember about institutional placement when counseling dementia patients and their families

1. Most of the public has a negative reaction to the idea of a nursing home, based on collective societal impressions about what they are like and the actual horrors exposed in the nursing home scandals of the 1960s and 1970s. Family members visualize them as places of squalor and suffering where their parent or relative will be neglected, or worse, abused. Each facility must be judged on its own merits, preferably after a personal visit and tour. Families should be helped in counseling to examine real alternatives about institutional care, and, encouraged to investigate possibilities on a firsthand basis. Some family members will be reluctant to go inside a nursing home to visit, and might need to be accompanied by the counselor or another professional with expertise in long-term care to provide technical advice and assistance with strong feelings that can be evoked during a visit. People who work in long-term care facilities become habituated to the sounds, sights of old, ailing people, smells, mood, and other environmental qualities that are so different from where most people spend their time. It can be a shock to enter a nursing home for the first time, not only because of the environmental qualities encountered but because a person who enters is confronted with the internal question, "What if I end up like they are, in a place like this?" Feelings about one's own aging, physical health, and care-giving network are easily aroused when inside a nursing home.

Families of dementia patients are usually further troubled about skilled level nursing homes because their demented relative is probably much more intact physically than the majority of the nursing home's residents. This may lead them to believe that their relative will be out of place, have nobody to spend time with, and in many other ways bear the ill effects of not "belonging with those other people." Such a realization is of course a tacit recognition of the problem with medical model nursing homes as a site for the care of dementia patients. Demented people in need of placement typically require extensive assistance with activities of daily living, psychosocial opportunities (sociocultural, interpersonal, creative, and symbolic-spiritual levels of need,[23] in addition to biological level needs (especially protection) while they are ambulatory and physically healthy. In contrast, most residents of skilled nursing facilities are physically incapacitated or bedridden with chronic illnesses, and many of these are likely to have some cognitive impairment[24] as well. Until there are a wider range of options at the intermediate care level and other less-skilled levels of the long-term care system, counseling will have to be oriented towards helping families cope with their frustration and persevering in their search for the best available option(s). In the meantime, advocacy effort directed toward developing and funding the "biopsychosocial" care[25] Alzheimer's and other demented patients need will continue.

2. Some families will reject nursing-home placement as an option for reasons based not on objective evidence, but on equally valid and important subjective feelings. They may be constrained by an overt or covert agreement, a "contract" of sorts made many years prior to any physical illness or dementia which was worded: "Promise me you'll never put me into a nursing home." These promises have usually been made with the assistance of denial ("Nothing will happen to my mother. She'll never get sick"), exploiting the need to please ("Tell me you'll never do anything I wouldn't approve of"), the need to set an example for the next generation ("I hope my children will see what I've done and use it as an example of what you should do for your parents"), and the collection of debts owed by the next generation ("I took care of my mother at home, and I expect my daughter to do the same for me").

Other emotional reasons for rejecting placement include the desire not to appear uncaring to friends, relatives, and neighbors, the need to demonstrate a continued or newfound devotion to the relative even when it is inviting martyrdom to do so,[26] and an inability to accept the reality of how the sickness or disability of the relative places both him/her and the family in jeopardy when reliable, good quality community-based care is absent. All of these reasons are valid and should be dealt with carefully in counseling. Utilizing the nine-step counseling model will, in many cases, help the family members clarify feelings and the demands of his/her conscience and rethink current options. But this in no way suggests that placement choices are easily resolved once emotions are confronted. Families faced with alternatives such as inadequate home care and substandard institutional care have no "good" choice and are often left feeling helpless, guilty, and depressed. Sometimes these situations will only permit the counselor to help the family accept that they did the best they could in spite of desires to have been able to do better.

3. People think of nursing homes as one step removed from the grave. Accepting the reality of placement can produce significant psychological changes once thought to be the result of institutionalization,[27] including demoralization, depression, apathy, and withdrawal. The overwhelming majority of people who enter a nursing home these days will likely live nowhere else except for brief hospital stays. Resistance to the idea of placement can therefore be viewed as an attempt to forestall an appointment with death. Good counseling technique advises that this aspect of the care-giver/families' emotional life be dealt with as an issue inherent in some families' reactions to the notion of nursing-home placement.

4. Even the best nursing homes are not *home,* and many older persons, demented or not, have trouble with the transition. For a demented person, placement can feel like a total abandonment by the family into a world that bears little resemblance to the one he/she just left. The memory impairment of the dementia patient makes it difficult to discuss the move with them, though some individuals can comprehend and retain some of what is going on. Patients will often ask, "Did I do something wrong?" or say, "You're not happy with me. I'll change what I'm doing, then can I stay?" when the subject is broached. Some patients evoke guilt by asking their children, "I don't understand why you're throwing me out. I can still live here, it's my home. Did I ever throw you out?" Others deny that any problem exists and respond to examples of memory loss, inappropriate behavior, or need for supervision by saying, "None of that is true. You're inventing it."

The counselor can help families focus on their experiences with the patient that demonstrate how impaired he/she is, and on the need for placement rather than persistently tuning in to their guilt and wishes that the patient's perceptions were correct and that there was no problem. Feelings that are real ("I feel like I'm letting mother down" or "I wish I didn't have to do this") can be separated from the family's need to deny painful realities ("Her memory is so bad that she really is a full-time job"). The counselor may say, "Being home alone while you both are out at work is not beneficial to her. She will do better with more assistance and stimulation." Such intervention can ease the guilt of care-givers and help them view what they have done as being the best of some imperfect choices.

Families often need support during their transition period to contend with their guilt, grief, and the patient's possible rejection or forgetting of them. It is not unusual for families to feel that they are "being punished" by the patient when he/she does not respond to them as before. While the patient may be feeling some anger the object of which cannot be pinpointed due to cognitive impairment, it is more likely that the demented person is simply showing evidence of living in the present. That is, he/she is relating most intensely to the new care-giver on whom he/she must rely. Former care-givers are responded to as familiar, loved people even if the specific name of their relationship cannot be articulated. This can cause hurt feelings. One child said: "I ask my mother who I am and she can't tell me. She just says I'm a nice lady. How can she forget that I'm her daughter?" Another laments: "She says I'm her mother! Can you believe that?" In this instance, the daughter is more likely to get the response she wants if she identifies herself to her mother, since her mother cannot perform the complex cognitive operation of identifying her face, and searching her memory for its referent. Determining which category of person, (relative, friend, neighbor, etc.) the individual belongs to, and choosing the right subcategory i.e., relative, friend, parent, child is a sophisticated mental act that is impaired by dementia. Some demented people develop an adaptive, universal response such as "I think we've met before" or "You look familiar." Counselors can help family members with these difficult times by: (1) helping the relative cope with feelings of rejection which accompany nonrecognition; (2) providing information about why misidentification or lack of recognition takes place; and (3) working on improved communication techniques so that the relative and patient can achieve optimal interaction even in the face of significant cognitive deficits.

Placement can be a difficult problem for the patient and the family, and there are no surefire ways to prevent difficulties from occurring. If the best possible match has been made between the patient's needs and the facilities resources, relative and patient will only have to contend with the problems of letting go and turning the care responsibilities over to somebody else. This process takes time and occasionally requires some counseling for those family members who can be overly critical or omnipresent as a way of demonstrating that nobody can care for their parent as well as they did. Patients can pick up such messages and resist becoming attached to the facility and its personnel for fear of offending their relative or in anticipation of leaving and returning to the care of that family member.

Such dynamics are often encountered in facilities and may begin as refusals to eat or participate, not unpacking, or constantly repacking one's belongings "to go home." This noninvolvement can also happen to patients attending day-treatment or other community-based programs, as can the family care-giver's conflict about letting go.[28] Counseling the family and the patients can produce benefits in both care environments.

If counselors are informed about the criteria for evaluating the quality of long term care,[29] they can help families take an active role in selecting a nursing home or other residential option. The best option will be the setting that treats the individuality of the demented individual as a positive basis for programming and care provision,[30] rather than as a thorn in the side of the staff. Families feel better about placing their relative if conditions exist that permit the patient to flourish; maintaining individuality is an essential part of this process. Counseling can then provide further assistance in finding institutions with good specialized innovative programs for people with dementia,[31] and in coping with the many feelings and conflicts that arise at this time in a family's life.

Appendix A

Alzheimer's and Other Dementias

Alzheimer's disease is but one of a number of conditions that are collectively called *dementias*. These are disorders that cause major behavioral changes in cognitive or intellectual abilities, and the adaptive behaviors that rely on these skills for their performance. In order for a person to be presumed to have a dementia, he/she must manifest a *global syndrome* involving a loss of mental abilities that interferes with the capacity to remember, think abstractly, use appropriate social skills and judgment, understand and produce spoken and written language, and work productively.

Dementia may also produce an alteration in personality in which the "real person" either changes noticeably (e.g., persons who have been nonaggressive become easily enraged) or manifests an accentuation of previously evident but nondominant personality traits. It is essential to bear in mind that dementia involves a collection (though not necessarily all) of these behaviors rather than one symptom in isolation as would be the case in aphasia (impairment of language ability) or personality disintegration, each of which can appear as a singular disorder. That is why dementia is referred to as a global disorder, and should not be considered as a possible diagnosis if only one symptom is present.

Symptoms of dementia vary in how disturbing they are to the victim and those around him/her. They also vary with regard to the pattern of symptom presentation. Below is a brief description of some of the typical manifestations of dementia that effect the behavioral capacities of the individual and that can produce great distress to the victim and family members. Some victims, however, manifest no conscious awareness of their symptoms and resist intervention despite cognitive dysfunction that is very apparent.

Dementias can occur at all ages of adult life, though they are more frequently seen and occur at an accelerating rate in people past the age of forty. People over the age of sixty-five constitute the vast majority of dementia patients, and seem to be by far the most well represented age group among Alzheimer's disease and multi-infarct dementia patients and their care-givers. It is therefore almost automatic to think of dementia as an older person's problem. It is an unfortunate problem that older people's increased risk for dementia is a consequence of the reduced death rate among the very old,[1] and that the incidence of dementias increases significantly with chronological age well into the eighth decade of life.[2] The incidence of Alzheimer's disease, the central subject of this book, increases with age, and while there are significant numbers of people under age sixty-five with Alzheimer's disease, the vast majority of persons with Alzheimer's and related disorders are in their sixties, seventies, and eighties.

Cognitive Symptoms of Dementia[3]

(A) *Memory impairment.* This is progressive and is more serious than occasionally forgetting where an item was left or someone's telephone number. A person with Alzheimer's dementia gradually becomes unable to remember current information (due to failing short-term memory) and progresses to being unable to remember how to get home or the name of a familiar relative. (Other dementias however can involve a loss of remote memory that occurs while recent memory remains relatively intact.) Ultimately the person has no functional memory, and lives only in the present.

(B) *Language impairment.* In progressive dementias language skills deteriorate over time. Called aphasia, this disability involves an inability to speak or write or to understand verbal or written messages. Specific language skills, such as the ability to name things, to construct sentences, to follow verbal or written directions, and to read or write are gradually lost. A demented person will often be able to read instructions aloud but not be able to carry them out properly. As language skills deteriorate, utterances lose complexity and accuracy with regard to grammar and syntax, and are thus more difficult to understand. Active vocabulary diminishes. A few retained words come to be used whenever a particular part of speech is required. Mrs. Humphrey says "bumpers" when she appears to want to say "clothes," "chair," or "people." Such communication impairment often proves to be very frustrating for care-givers and victims alike, and can even become dangerous if the victim is unable to express the presence or location of physical pain, feelings of hunger or thirst, and other discomfort.

(C) *Inability to perform purposeful movement.* Self-care capability relies on our brain's ability to select an appropriate response in a given stimulus environment and, given no physical impairment, execute it at the appropriate time. Eating with utensils at the dinner table, or putting clothes on with buttons buttoned and zippers zipped are examples of this complex skill. The inability to perform such purposeful acts is called apraxia, and occurs in progressive dementias with increasing severity over time. What starts out as the inability to button a sweater or walk briskly without tripping becomes the inability to step into shoes, sit on the toilet without verbal (and later physical) assistance, or ultimately to walk at all. As apraxia progresses, the daily care functions of the person must be partially and later totally assumed by a care-giver.

(D) *Perceptual impairment.* In order to comprehend the meaning of an object or any other sensory stimulus, a person must first have intact sensory capacities (e.g., vision, hearing, smell, etc.) and then must process the sensory information to recognize or match it to prior stimuli that it resembles. Agnosia, the inability to know or understand the meaning of sensory information, characterizes victims of dementia who typically develop tendencies to misidentify objects (e.g., they eat plants or urinate in the wastebasket). Dementia renders items in the environment increasingly less recognizable as discreet objects with particular functions or uses. They become increasingly responded to with best and largely inappropriate "guesstimates" as to their meaning and functions. People are misidentified as well, or are told that they are not who they say they are. An example of agnosia is illustrated in the following dialogue. The patient, an eighty-two-year-old man with Alzheimer's dementia named Martin Smith, Sr., was accompanied by his son, Martin, Jr., age fifty-seven.

Dialogue:

COUNSELOR: Can you tell me your name?
MR. SMITH: Martin A. Smith.
COUNSELOR: Good. Now can you tell me who is sitting in the chair across from you? (i.e., his son)
MR. SMITH: No, who is he?
COUNSELOR: Have you seen him before?
MR. SMITH: No, I don't think I have, but I am glad to know him. (*To the son*) Glad to know you.
COUNSELOR: Since you say you don't know him, I'll tell you that he has the same name as you.
MR. SMITH: Really. Is that so? What a thing, it's a real coincidence!
COUNSELOR: His name is Martin A. Smith, Jr. Do you know who that might be?
MR. SMITH: Really, is that his name?
COUNSELOR: Yes, can you tell me if he's any relation to you?
MR. SMITH: I don't think he is.
COUNSELOR: Mr. Smith, that man is your son.
MR. SMITH: No! That can't be, my son is ten years old.

The senior Mr. Smith had undergone a memory loss such that he could not recall any evidence that his son was past ten years old. Therefore, that fifty-seven-year-old could not be matched to any memory trace Mr. Smith had available so as to define who that grown man was.

(E) *Learning ability.* Due largely to the impairment of short-term memory found in dementia, the ability to encode new information and store it in memory is lost. It is therefore difficult for most dementia victims, notably those with Alzheimer's disease, to become familiar with new stimuli and thereby keep every situation from being totally new and unconnected to previous experiences. It may be the difficulty of recognizing a new living environment, a new grandchild, new routines, or other such problem that is the cause for concern in a person with dementia or his/her family. This diminution of learning ability transforms the world of the demented person from a relatively secure world of patterns, predictability, and regularity into a world of surprises, randomness, and anxiety. In many dementias, particularly Alzheimer's disease and multi-infarct dementias, some learning ability is retained at the early stages of the disorders. Remediation through the use of memory training and the like is therefore a worthwhile undertaking.

(F) *Disorientation.* Knowing the place, time, and whom one is with are necessary skills if a person is to display behavioral congruence with those around him/her. Persons with dementia lose the ability to identify correctly the day, date, year, location, and are unable to name those who are around them. This can occur gradually as in Alzheimer's disease, or suddenly for a number of other reasons, such as multiple infarcts or acute physical illnesses.

(G) *Personality changes.* Persons with dementia may manifest personality changes that can become the most distressing symptom to family members. Once sedate, refined, church-going ladies begin to utter obscenities that would make even the most hardened construction worker blush. Proper gentlemen have been reported to become sexually disinhibited and make sexual advances to strange women. Most typically, however, people who never got overtly angry may begin to become enraged for no apparent reason, and may even become physically and/or verbally abusive. These changes are usually reported by family members who say, "This is not my father." Major outbursts of rage over minor matters are called "catastrophic reactions." These episodes can prove to be very embarrassing to the patient and to witnesses of these episodes, especially the family. This behavior is thought to be the result of the brain deterioration causing the dementia and is apparently not under the control of the patient.

(H) *Wandering.* This term is used to refer to the patient's moving about "in a seemingly aimless disoriented fashion, or in pursuit of an indefinable or unobtainable goal."[4] In wandering, a person with dementia walks out of the door to his/her home and when asked for his/her destination replies, "I'm going home." Upon being told, "You are home, you live here. This is your house, and has been for thirty years," the person might reply, "No it isn't, and I'm going to walk home." Other forms of wandering include walking up and down the halls of an institution or walking endlessly through the house.

(I) *Suspicion, delusions, and paranoia.* Another disturbing symptom found in some demented people is a severe distrust of the motives of formerly trusted relatives or friends, even to the point of believing that people are plotting to harm them or steal their possessions. Delusions are fixed ideas with no basis in fact, such as that one's behavior is being controlled by people sending radio waves from across town.

(J) *Hallucinations and misinterpretations.* Hallucinations are very alarming symptoms because they raise the specter of craziness and impairment severe enough to require psychiatric hospitalization. These sensory experiences for which there are no objectively observable stimuli also produce fear responses in care-givers. Auditory and visual hallucinations may become dangerous because the person may physically respond to what the voices are telling him to do or to visual threats of danger. Misinterpretations, often called illusions, result from a misunderstanding of experiences and a misinterpretation of events or misidentification of people. An example of such a phenomenon would be when a demented man insists that his spouse is his mother or sister, or when a demented person becomes fearful upon hearing care-givers talk angrily about someone else and thinks they are angry at her.

These misinterpretations occur when a demented person sees or hears fragmentary information in the environment and constructs a mental explanation of events based on his/her faulty mental ability.

Case Example

Mrs. Porter lived in a nursing home and in spite of her moderate dementia, read a newspaper every day. While she could understand what she read, she would personalize events she read about and believe a relative of hers was the subject of the news stories. Each afternoon she'd get very agitated and say, "I have to get out of here. Something terrible has happened to my family." An alert staff was able to check the newspaper Mrs. Porter had read lately and determined that she was personalizing these stories of plane crashes, auto accidents, etc., as she encoded them into memory, and was probably "filling in the gaps" of information with her own emotional reality. That is, she had not "seen" her family for a long time (actually not the case—they visited frequently but her lack of short-term memory made it seem as though they had vanished forever when they were not actually present) and presumed that these accidents were the reason why.

Miss Collins is demented to a moderate degree yet lives at home with full-time care. She watches television a great deal and believes that the action on the screen is actually taking place in her room or just outside her home.

These are just some of the behavioral disturbances that may be present in dementias of various kinds. They are not exclusive to Alzheimer's disease, or any other, and are not diagnostic of one dementia or another. They are, however, illustrative of the wide variety of disturbing behaviors that make up the global impairments of cognition called dementia.

Dementias are usually characterized according to their age at onset, that is, do they begin before or after age sixty-five, and their reversibility. In the past it was customary to speak of acute vs. chronic dementia, which were typically referred to as "Organic Brain Syndrome." This led to many unfortunate, erroneous, self-fulfilling prophecies in which the diagnosis and hence the future course of a dementia patient were all too often decided largely on the basis of the patient's age. Many older people with potentially reversible dementias were labeled as having "chronic" and presumably untreatable conditions simply by virtue of being old and disoriented or confused. Up until the late 1970s and early 1980s there were unfortunately and tragically many old people so diagnosed who were needlessly condemned to lives of hopelessness and deterioration as once reversible dementias were left untreated and indeed did become chronic or fatal. Greater awareness, improved diagnostic techniques and acumen available in the professional community, and a more sophisticated and informed public have reduced— though by no means eliminated—such nihilism and unnecessary mental impairments in our older population. We therefore will consider dementias with a view toward those that are potentially reversible and those that are not. While the dementias due to normal pressure hydrocephalus or diabetes, for example, can be successfully reversed by surgery in the former case and diet or medication in the latter, not all individuals are good candidates for surgery, (the older they are the higher the mortality risk) or will remain easily under control with insulin or diet.[5]

Age at onset is another category used to classify dementias. Sixty-five is chosen as somewhat of an arbitrary dividing line, though there is nothing magical that happens at age sixty-five in all persons to make this age a threshold to cognitive impairment. The age at onset is probably most useful as an indicator of the kinds of psychosocial stresses caused by dementia to the patient and family. "Early onset" (before age sixty-five) and "late onset" (after sixty-five) are commonly used distinctions.

Potentially reversible dementias.

Raskind and Storrie[6] and Roth[7] describe some of the frequently seen causes of potentially reversible dementias in older persons. These include:

Toxic reactions to: Barbiturate use, alcoholism, multiple drug usage (prescribed and over-the-counter).

Metabolic disorders: e.g., potassium loss can be a result of diuretic usage or self-purgation also sodium, chloride or other electrolyte imbalance, hypercalcemia, mercury, or lead toxicity.

Nutritional disorders: Poor nutrition (especially when person is isolated and self-neglectful), vitamin B_{12} deficiency, (pernicious anemia), folic acid deficiency.

Infection: Pulmonary tuberculosis, bacterial endocarditis, chronic respiratory infection, chronic urinary tract infection.

Systemic illness or disorders: Congestive heart failure and/or low cardiac output states, diseases of lung, kidney, liver, thyroid, parathyroid, pituitary glands, diabetes, or hypoglycemia.

Structural causes: Slowly growing cerebral tumor, meningiomas, normal pressure hydrocephalus, subdural hematoma.

Nonreversible dementias:

Nonreversible dementias are primarily due to Alzheimer's disease, multi-infarct dementia, a combination of both (mixed dementia), other less frequently occurring disorders, and for causes as yet unknown. The list below outlines some of these.

Nonreversible dementias can be due to:

1. Alzheimer's disease.
2. Multiple infarcts and other vascular origins.
3. Parkinson's disease.
4. Progressive supranuclear palsy.
5. Huntington's disease.
6. Multiple sclerosis.
7. AIDS.
8. Other infectious, transmittable origins such as Creutzfeldt-Jakob disease, syphilis, or kuru.
9. Down's syndrome.
10. Pick's disease.
11. Wernicke's encephalopathy leading (in eighty percent of cases) to Korsakoff's syndrome (found frequently among alcoholics).
12. Idiopathic causes unknown or no abnormal physical findings found on autopsy in spite of observable dementia.

A full discussion of these conditions is not possible here. The interested reader is referred to relevant and more comprehensive literature listed at the end of this book. Despite differences in some symptoms and the physical basis of each disorder, we can address our remarks about counseling and dealing with the people involved to dementia victims in general regardless of a specific diagnosis. No matter the ultimate source of the neuronal devastation and cognitive impairment, people faced with progressive, irreversible conditions such as these require an intervention approach that goes beyond their diagnostic label and touches their humanness.

These conditions have been presented at this point so that the reader might become familiar with the many disorders that can cause reversible and nonreversible dementias in later life, and so that the complexity of diagnosing the cause(s) of dementia can begin to be understood. This is an especially complex issue, since a person can have more than one dementia at a time. In fact it is not unusual for a nonreversible dementia to be complicated by another reversible or nonreversible one (e.g., mixed Alzheimer's dementia and multi-infarct dementia, or Alzheimer's dementia with an acute drug toxicity, chronic infection and/or diabetes). Having Alzheimer's disease unfortunately does not rule out further impairments of cognitive functions by another dementia, though it can result in the lack of further diagnostic investigations or treatment for the secondary dementing condition.

Delirium

A condition of global cognitive impairment with a disturbance in the state of consciousness and associated attention difficulties (e.g., lethargy or hyperexcitability) is called delirium. Such a condition is due to organic disturbances that typically lead to the rapid onset of memory impairment and disorientation, and a fluctuating attention level. Other symptoms include perceptual disturbances (misinterpretation of environmental stimuli, or hallucinations) incoherent speech, reduced wakefulness or insomnia, and increases or decreases in motoric activity (restlessness or motor retardation).

The attentional deficit seen in delirium makes evaluation and treatment problematic. The person cannot pay attention for any length of time, and cannot think about goal-directed behavior or perform goal-oriented actions. In contrast to dementia, disorders of memory and orientation are secondary rather than primary.[8] Because the patient cannot attend to stimuli, he or she is unable to register and retain new information. An episode of delirium can last from one hour to a few days. Attendant fluctuations in lucidity can lead to confusion and disagreement among observers as to what is actually happening. Delirium can co-occur with dementia(s), and it is not uncommon to reverse a delirium by appropriate therapy and find dementia. Causes of delirium are numerous and are in many instances the same as the factors implicated in reversible dementias. The major categories of precipitants to delirium include:

Drug toxicity: digitalis, antiparkinsonian drugs, corticosteroids, psychotropic medications such as tricyclic antidepressants, and so called "major" and "minor" tranquilizers.

Neurologic disorders: head trauma, cerebrovascular accidents, seizures, meningitis.

Systemic illness: congestive heart failure, liver, kidney, or lung insufficency, infection, burns, lupus erythematosus.

Metabolic disorders: thyroid disorder, hypoglycemia, elevated calcium levels secondary to calcium resorbtion or antacid misuse.

Postoperative status: slower excretion of anesthetic by older persons.

Withdrawal from: alcohol, sedatives or hypnotics.[9]

Treatment of delirium requires that the underlying organic problem be dealt with, typically in a medical setting. Only after this has been successfully accomplished can "talking therapies" or counseling be undertaken.

Depression

One of the more difficult diagnostic decisions to be made by a clinician concerns the differentiation between Alzheimer's and related dementias and the cognitive impairments that accompany depression. This is a particularly crucial distinction since depression is a treatable disorder that may produce cognitive impairment. If left untreated, depression can lead to worsening dementia resulting from malnutrition, physical danger due to confusion and disorientation, greatly reduced quality of life due to sadness and hopelessness, and if severe enough, suicidal thought or action.

Depression can occur in the elderly for different reasons. It can be a lifelong personality component with which the person has aged, or it can be a reaction to a real or feared loss (e.g., the death of a spouse or the loss of physical capacity or role relationship) occurring in later life. Depression can also be present in the so called "two-tiered" variety. In this instance an individual with a depressive personality reacts with depression to significant losses or suffers one of the other etiologies of depression.

Depressive disorders usually (though not always) are signaled by: sad, tearful affect, physical symptoms such as aches and pains (often the early complaint), early awakening from a night's sleep, poor appetite and resultant weight loss, decreased libido, unexplained fatigue, and constipation or urinary difficulties. The person may manifest psychomotor retardation, i.e., slowness of speech, thought, gait and physical action, or, conversely, agitation. Hopelessness, helplessness, irritability, "decisional impotence," chronic dissatisfaction, emptiness, feelings of worthlessness and uselessness, suicidal ideas, or verbalization and memory disturbances are other frequently seen symptoms. Some "memory loss" occurs in depressed people because they are focused inward and are not in tune with their external environment, so that external stimuli are not perceived, encoded, stored, or retrievable. This renders the person memory-impaired; though in fact he/she may never have taken in any information to remember. Many observers report that depressed patients appear to have a memory loss based on a loss of will to remember or lack of energy to conduct the search through the mental memory banks. "I don't know" is a frequent answer to questions of orientation and information, though this may not be a foolproof sign of cognitive impairment due to depression in dementia of other origins.[10] Many older, depressed people will display mainly hypochondriacal complaints and have few other symptoms of depression; others will have vague memory complaints.

Unlike the progressive onset of Alzheimer's disease or other gradual onset dementias where memory loss is typically attested to by retrospective family data, the cognitive dysfunction in depression has an identifiable date of onset, which can usually be located in the recent (thirty to sixty days) past. In such cases it is helpful to look for recent losses, physical illnesses, drug introduction or prolonged utilization or dosage change, (especially digitalis, "major" or "minor" tranquilizers, alcohol, antiparkinsonian drugs, cardiac medicines containing reserpine, and others) as possible etiological factors.[11] Proper diagnostic intervention is vital due to the above-mentioned suicide risk and because of the fear of senility that older persons have to make them avoid professional attention lest their fears be confirmed.

A gross differentiation between depression-related cognitive dysfunction and possible Alzheimer's or related disorder can be tentatively made with reference to the differences listed below.[12]

Possible Depression	*Possible Dementias*
1. Complaints exceed actual impairment	Impairment minimized
2. Depression persists	Affect labile and shallow
3. Complains about self and focuses on failure	Denies problems or blames others
4. Delusions are congruent with depressed mood	Delusions are shallow
5. Relatively sudden with identifiable time of onset	Insidious (except multi-infarct) with no clear date of onset
6. Rapid cognitive deterioration with recent onset	Gradual deterioration (except step-wise in multi-infarct)
7. Memory improves as depression gets better	Improves temporarily if at all

8. Can find way around and knows whom to ask for help   Gets lost in familiar environment; asks anyone for help
9. May be worse in A.M., better in P.M.   May be better in A.M.; deteriorates as day goes on

Why Is Accurate Diagnosis Vital?

Precisely because the myth of senility is untrue, it is important that any older person who experiences loss of memory, confusion about the date, time, location, people's names, inability to calculate, be treated as a person with a serious condition which is not normal.

The possibility that the cognitive disorder is potentially reversible makes it even more imperative that the underlying cause(s) be found and treated. Given what is known about the origins of cognitive disturbances in the elderly, it is no longer acceptable to have these shrugged off as inevitable, untreatable senility that is to be expected and accepted simply due to a person's chronological age.

In early stages it can be difficult to differentiate cognitive dysfunction due to depression from Alzheimer's dementia. More than likely if the affected individual is a victim of Alzheimer's disease he/she may also respond to it with a reactive depression.

Because this sequence of events is disturbingly common, a proper diagnostic workup as to the cause (if identifiable) of the cognitive impairment is vital. The following is the generally accepted method to try to find a specific cause and, hopefully, a treatment.

Diagnostic Evaluation of Dementia[13]

1. Personal and medical history from patient if possible and a family member, care-giver, friend, or other informed source.
2. Psychiatric evaluation, mental status exam, psychiatric history (if any) especially to rule out chronic schizophrenia, bipolar disorder, depression (reactive).
3. Medical evaluation: medication inventory; complete physical; electrocardiogram; complete blood count; urinalysis; urine toxicology screen; blood tests for VDRL (syphilis), bromide level, sodium, potassium, chloride, calcium levels, measures of liver and kidney functions, blood glucose levels; chest X ray, CAT scan of the head (to rule out tumors and to identify evidence of old infarcts or other insults), cerebral blood flow, Vitamin B_{12} and Folic acid level, thyroid studies.
4. Neurological evaluation, to rule out, e.g.: Parkinson's disease, progressive supranuclear palsy, Huntington's disease, normal pressure hydro-

cephalus, and others.
5. Neuropsychological evaluation; to further clarify the nature of the disorder, assess degree of impairment, and prescribe compensatory intervention strategies.

If this exhaustive evaluation fails to identify another specific basis for the patient's cognitive impairment, it is presumable though not certain that Alzheimer's disease may be the source of the impairment. No single test listed above will yield results diagnostic of Alzheimer's disease, and in fact Alzheimer's disease has no known "marker" that differentiates it from other dementias while the person is alive. Some promising work on the course and patterns of behavioral change in Alzheimer's dementia is being done, but it is not yet universally used as a diagnostic index. A recent report on the differential diagnosis of dementing diseases provides the most current guidelines recommended by national experts.[14]

Alzheimer's Disease

Senile dementia of the Alzheimer's type (SDAT) is the most frequently seen basis of nonreversible cognitive disability in persons sixty-five years of age and older. Alzheimer's disease accounts for fifty to sixty-five percent of these dementias.[15] In real numbers, this means that around 2.5 to 6 million people are affected by Alzheimer's type dementia. (Estimates vary due to problems of diagnostic accuracy in samples used and the lack of positive diagnostic organic signs until an autopsy is obtainable.) Another twelve to sixteen percent are victims of *multi-infarct dementia* (due to blood clots in small vessels of the brain), making it the second most common cause of irreversible dementia. Autopsy studies have found that the damage to the brain in this dementia is due to small-vessel damage and not cerebral arteriosclerosis or large-vessel narrowing as was previously believed. Multi-infarct dementia is treatable to a degree, but is nonetheless a progressive dementia.

What then is the cause of Alzheimer's disease? In reality, nobody really knows why this disease occurs, and therefore no cure is yet available. There are a number of theories as to the etiology of Alzheimer's disease and many of these theories are under active investigation. Leading candidates for causation include a slow-acting virus, genetic factors, immunological defects, toxins (e.g., aluminum), or combinations of some of these. It has been observed that people with Alzheimer's disease are significantly lacking in a substance called choline acetyltransferase, an enzyme needed for the neurotransmission that allows short-term memory to occur. (Neurotransmitters are biochemical substances found between dendrites, the hairlike ends of nerve cells, which act as bridges to facilitate the transfer of a nervous impulse from one cell to a contiguous one.) It also appears that people with Alzheimer's disease have fewer cells in their brain in which acetylcholine appears to be manufactured (the substance from which choline acetyltransferase is made). Results have so far not demonstrated any significant replicable benefits of dietary or pharmacological therapies to supplement shortages of acetylcholine in Alzheimer's-disease patients.

Though its cause(s) are unknown, there appear to be characteristic pathological changes in the brains of most victims of Alzheimer's disease. These alterations of the configuration of nerve cells seen under the microscope were first described by Dr. Alois Alzheimer in 1907. He observed the gradual intellectual deterioration of a woman in her early fifties whose husband reported that she had become progressively forgetful, suspicious, and less able to care for herself. After the patient died, Alzheimer examined the cells of her brain under a microscope. He found *neuritic plaques* and *neurofibrillary tangles*, the phenomena that have come to be regarded as telltale (though not conclusive) evidence of Alzheimer's disease. What is significant about these neuritic plaques and neurofibrillary tangles is that they provide physical evidence that the brain is indeed damaged and that they occur in Alzheimer's victims in far greater profusion than they do in nondemented persons of the same age. Thus, the behavior must be viewed as due to underlying brain pathology and not "normal aging" or negativism. In a most significant investigation, Blessed et al[16] were able to demonstrate a significant positive relationship between the profusion of these neuropathological markers found on autopsy and the extent of demented behavior while the person was alive. Finally, the evidence of these brain changes in Alzheimer's-disease victims identifies a different physical basis for the disorder than the dementias of vascular origin (e.g., multi-infarct dementia), which can have a different symptom picture and clinical course as well.

While the search for the cause(s) and hopefully the eventual cure(s) proceeds, the lives of Alzheimer's-disease victims and their families continue to be adversely effected by the behavior and personal erosion brought on by the disease. Interventions in the form of various treatment options are currently being developed.

Since Alzheimer's disease is a progressive dementia—that is, its symptoms appear in a gradual, slow progression over a number of years—it is important to be aware of the pattern(s) of onset of the disorder. This is vital not only because it appears that Alzheimer's disease may have a characteristic course[17] that may aid in diagnosis, but because intervention goals will differ according to biopsychosocial needs and capabilities of the victims (and families) as the disease progresses. Sufficient observations of large numbers of SDAT victims have been made so that we can currently utilize global descriptions of behavioral phases of the disorder to orient our thinking and perhaps categorize service and intervention requirements. A cautionary note is in order here, since there is a great degree of individual difference in how persons with SDAT behave. These individual patterns are critical foci for any intervention efforts. The impact of the disease on cognitive ability is not uniform. Depending on how much deterioration has occurred and its particular location in each area of the brain (i.e., what the course of each disease process is), patients will display different symptom pictures. Indeed, these frequently are the bases of differential diagnosis. People vary in their response to each symptom as well. Further complications to a complete, universal "stage" description of SDAT are introduced by the effects of other illnesses and/or dementias that complicate the clinical picture and the effects of drugs on the person's behavior and cognitive capacity. Thus it cannot be presumed that all cognitive dysfunction seen in any given victim of SDAT is due entirely to the neurodegenerative effects of Alzheimer's disease. By the same token, it cannot be correctly presumed that all Alzheimer's patients in the same phase will behave identically or respond equally well to the same treatment.

Nevertheless, we have available to us some helpful guidelines as to constellations of cognitive dysfunctions that tend to occur in a characteristic sequence. These phases are not without variation, however. The behavioral descriptions are drawn from the work of Lisa Gwyther[18] and material published by the Burke Rehabilitation Center.[19]

Phases of SDAT Dysfunction

First phase

- The person loses spontaneity and energy for life
- Is more easily angered
- Is slow to react to stimuli, and picks up new information more slowly and with greater number of errors
- Shows less initiative and greater reluctance to undertake new activities
- Will stick with familiar, patterned or predictable activities or actions
- May take longer with routine chores
- Finds him/herself unable to think of words, especially names of things, people, or places
- Loses the way going to a familiar place
- Has trouble in handling money, paying bills, regulating financial affairs (e.g., balancing checkbook)
- Gets anxious or withdrawn—"I feel foolish"

Dynamics: In this phase, it becomes evident that the person cannot do things as well as he/she once did, especially in social and interpersonal spheres. People who were "thinkers" experience loss of self-esteem as intellectual capacity declines and may attempt to "cover" symptoms. Logical thinking remains but recent memory is impaired, so the person can invent reasons why his/her errors in judgment and decisions are not unreasonable. Disagreements among family members are not uncommon because of this. Relatives and friends have evidence to see what they want to see and confirm their sense that Mom or Dad is "OK" or that "there is something wrong." Children also get into arguments with parents suspected of having cognitive impairments who typically use their intact logic and parental authority to deny all allegations of memory problems. The behaviors in this phase are frequently mistaken for signs of normal aging and maybe dismissed with the proverbial "What do you expect at my age?" Phase 1 behaviors are strikingly similar to early signs of depression in older people, and, since these are often assumed to be "normal aging," differential diagnosis is difficult without expert assessment. In both cases people are either consciously or unconsciously reacting to their "fear of senility" and engaging in rationalization and/or denial.

Examples:

1. Repeatedly loses things (not just occasionally).
2. Loses count in card games, can't keep score at golf, forgets often-dialed phone numbers.
3. Pays same bills many times or not at all. Can't balance the checkbook so the bank returns checks as unpaid. Utilities may be shut off for nonpayment.
4. Orders endlessly from door-to-door salesmen, catalogues, telephone solicitors, etc., at times because he/she has forgotten what was ordered, or because in a desire to appear "nice" the patient hides a lack of comprehension about the nature of the transaction by agreeing to anything.
5. Hides things so as "not to lose them" or to protect them from being "taken by others."
6. Makes a favorite dinner and forgets to prepare some courses.
7. Continually makes errors about appointments or location of places.

Second Phase

- Has problem recognizing familiar persons, e.g., relatives and friends.
- Has great difficulty with decisions, plans, and social encounters.
- Speech is noticeably slower and impoverished, with noticeable repetition of certain words or phases. Loses the thread of a story, though words are understandable.
- May make up stories (confabulate) to fill in empty spaces in memory.
- Has trouble comprehending what he/she reads.
- Can't write clearly, and is unable to calculate.

- Is more self-absorbed and loses the ability to understand how others feel.
- Late-afternoon restlessness ("Sundowner's Syndrome").
- Has difficulty with perceptual motor coordination, i.e., is unable to sit down in a chair without risk of missing it, can't shave self.
- Emotional disinhibition occurs; may be teary, angry, silly, or irritable without apparent external stimuli to trigger emotions. Acts impulsively.
- Loses the ability to maintain physical self without assistance. Will not bathe (or is afraid to).
- Cannot monitor status of physical appearance, so wears underclothes outside of slacks or shirt. Doesn't care about looking neat or "appropriate."
- Makes repetitive physical movements, e.g., tapping, walking, picking up imaginary lint or dust.
- May have sensory experience with no basis in objective reality (illusions or hallucinations).
- Cannot exist without some supervision (at onset of this phase) and ultimately needs total supervision (by the end).
- "Catastrophic" emotional reactions to seemingly minor events. Is easily overloaded by too many stimuli.

Dynamics: This phase, which lasts an average of anywhere from two to ten years, marks the obvious and undeniable transition from residual autonomy to dependency. The basic cognitive skills required to engage in higher-order thinking and engage in complex human activity deteriorate so much that abstract logic and linguistic ability are replaced with developmentally more primitive concrete thinking, lack of objectivity (egocentrism), and increased anxiety as the person becomes lost in an incomprehensible world. Interpersonal relationships are rooted in dependency-dependability issues, and many attempts at autonomy misfire horrendously. The historical balance between parents and children is reversed, so that parents become care-recipients and children care-providers—a shift often accompanied by great stress on both generations. Sadness and guilt are major difficulties as caring and potentially care-giving children or spouses must confront the gap between their long-held wishes and plans for the future and the realities of caring for a dementing relative. Embarrassing events occur with great frequency. The police may ring the doorbell to return a lost relative; a demented spouse may call the police to say that a strange person is living in the home and sleeping in his/her bed. In some social situations, persons exhibiting second-phase dementia syndrome will often respond to hallucinations or illusions and say, "I'm leaving, my father is waiting for me downtown" and walk out without a coat in a snowstorm. The person might eat with his/her fingers and do so noisily in a fine restaurant. Use of foul language and disrobing in public are other signs of behavioral breakdown, which cause great consternation for relatives and friends. These latter behaviors illustrate the disturbing impact of disinhibition and it is in this context that they should be understood rather than being labeled "childish behavior."

Examples:

1. Can't remember visitors immediately after they left.
2. Sleeps frequently, wakes up more disoriented, and gets ready to go to work.
3. Is unable to follow directions, though apparently understands them.
4. Uncertain about how to behave, so does nothing or withdraws from a situation.
5. Has virtually no recent memory, but good remote memory. Interprets recent events in context of the past as if they were current reality.
6. Memory is lost retrogressively, so points of orientation to time, place, and person are drawn from cues further and further back in experience and time.
7. Gets "lost" due to "unfamiliarity" of location (has forgotten it) and wanders to reorient self or calls for help to go home.
8. Suspiciousness may cause victim to blame others for his/her errors (such as misplacing things) or to accuse loved ones of harmful motives to explain current state of affairs.
9. Constantly tries to eat other people's food or craves "junk food."
10. Invents words (neologisms) and gets annoyed when listeners do not understand them.

Third Phase:

- Is apathetic, remote, and unable to recognize family or his/her own image in the mirror.
- Loses weight, in spite of an adequate diet.
- Recent memory and remote memory are poor.
- Cannot find his/her way around.
- Becomes incontinent of urine and feces.
- May put all objects into his/her mouth or touch them.
- Unable to communicate with words, and produces perseverative syllables, word fragments, or intonational vocalization with no semantic meaning but with emotional content.
- Can understand emotional messages and emotional tone of speech, though cannot speak.
- May experience seizures, skin breakdown if unable to move, and accelerating number of physical sequelae of immobilization.
- Cannot walk or move large muscles, may experience muscle contractions.

- Remains responsive in small ways to quality of physical care giving.

Dynamics: This "terminal stage," as it has been called, can last an average of one to three years and is the time when care needs become primarily physical, though emotional reassurance is critical. Care-givers often feel depleted from the lack of emotional feedback from the patient. The total physical care is particularly burdensome on family care-givers, who often give out under the stress of round-the-clock care demands experienced on any given day. It is not uncommon for the care-giving spouse to develop serious physical illness and even die as a result of the stress and strain involved with such care.

Examples:

1. If ambulatory, handles everything as a way of comprehending it or puts things in mouth again.
2. May need to be physically restrained if no supervision is available to prevent injury due to falls from exhaustion.
3. Person is unable to bathe, dress, eat, or go to the bathroom without help.
4. Makes sounds (phonation) that have no apparent meaning but can be annoying to listen to for long periods of time.

In summary, Alzheimer's disease is a progressive, chronic dementia that causes a gradual loss of mental abilities. It is the most common of the nonreversible dementias. The gradual steady decline of mentation shown by SDAT patients is associated with characteristic neuropathological changes throughout the brain usually found on autopsy. The slow, gradual pattern of deterioration is in contrast to the stepwise deterioration found with multi-infarct dementia, the second leading cause of nonreversible dementias.

The presence of SDAT in a person is presumed based on a diagnosis of exclusion as there is no specific test for it. Other causes of dementia (reversible and nonreversible) must be explored before SDAT is properly considered the diagnosis. This cannot be done by "eyeballing" a patient but must instead involve extensive testing and expert evaluations of various kinds. Delirium and depression are reversible conditions often mistakenly thought to be SDAT.

While there is no universally accepted "stage" description of SDAT, there are progressions that are characteristic of many SDAT victims. There is still no valid and reliable psychometric test battery that pinpoints Alzheimer's disease and excludes other causes of dementia. Individual differences, personality, complications of illness, drugs, and the specific location of nerve cell damage all play a part in how each patient appears to behave and the symptom picture at any point in the course of dementia.

Counseling Considerations

Avoidance and Denial:

People with changes in memory fear that they are getting "senile" (even young people). They therefore avoid finding out the cause because they are afraid it is "senility" or these days, Alzheimer's disease. Reassuring people that their memory problem might be a reversible disorder, especially if caught early, is an important intervention. One must be encouraging about the likelihood that the problem can be helped without reinforcing the patient's denial that nothing is really wrong. Nihilism must be confronted, both with professionals and families, as must the mistaken notion that memory impairments are "normal" at any older ages. Referral to a qualified professional or diagnostic center is crucial both to establish credibility of the diagnosis and to assure accuracy.

Counselors must also face the problems caused by friends and families not wanting to "upset" the person with cognitive impairment. The following case illustrates how this can cause family dissension and even potential danger:

Example:

Mrs. Brown's niece came to see her aunt and was startled to hear that this beloved relative had been leaving the stove on, forgot where she was in the middle of church services, and was unable to recognize her family at a fiftieth wedding anniversary party for her brother. Mrs. Brown's neighbors confided to the niece that this had been going on for about two years, but that it had become noticeably worse about two months prior to this visit. When Mrs. Brown's niece made an appointment to have her aunt's memory problem looked into, Mrs. Brown became angry, denied any memory problem, and demanded that her neighbors and friends tell her niece that nothing was wrong. Fearing that they would upset Mrs. Brown if they were truthful, they confirmed her denial. This lent validity to Mrs. Brown's suspicions that her niece was plotting to get her money by having her declared insane or incompetent. Mrs. Brown's condition worsened, and a month later the neighbors again called the niece and begged her to do something. The niece at this point asserted that their reinforcing of her aunt's denial was making it impossible to convince Mrs. Brown that there was any objective evidence for the problems they were reporting. One month later Mrs. Brown had a massive CVA (stroke) and died. It was likely that the recent memory changes observed by the neighbors and family were due to multi-infarct dementia.

Denial by patients and family members is quite understandable as a reaction to the (unconscious) recognition of symptoms, though this usually gives way to anger and other emotions. It has been suggested that patients are more likely to underestimate the severity of their memory problems, or deny them, and that family members are better able to estimate the severity of the patient's cognitive difficulty.[20] Their reaction to the actual diagnosis can include denial as well, since to recognize the full impact of what this disease will mean to the quality of their lives for the next five to twenty years (depending on how long the patient lives) is something not easily accomplished all at once. Forcing people to recognize unpleasant, even horrifying reality is not conducive to good adjustment; counseling in these circumstances must be oriented toward helping clients absorb as much as they can at any point and continuing to assist them as denial lessens.

If the members of a family choose to disbelieve the diagnosis of Alzheimer's disease, they are not behaving altogether unreasonably. After all, since there is no positive diagnosis available it can be possible that the diagnosis is an error. Wanting to obtain another opinion is an understandable reaction, and if circumstances and finances permit, this option should be explored.

Appendix B

Care Services for Dementia Patients

Adult Day-Care: Partial or all-day supervision; social, physical recreation, and/or therapeutic programs.

Case Management: Linkage, coordination, and assessment.

Chore Services: Assistance with home-care functions such as shopping, paying bills, doing errands.

Congregate Meals: Nutritionally supervised meals served in a setting that encourages social contact with others. Usually available for a suggested nominal contribution.

Dental Needs: Poor oral health may complicate overall wellness, exacerbate the problems in chewing or swallowing dementia patients experience as a result of their disease, and compromise nutritional adequacy. Particular care is needed for dementia patients who may panic, refuse to remain seated or to sit still, and who may become aggressive.

Home-delivered Meals: Usually require that the recipients be homebound.

Home Health Aide Service: Assists with bathing, feeding toileting, dressing, and other personal care, monitors physical integrity, provides reorientation if needed.

Homemaker Services: Cooking, cleaning, shopping.

Hospice Services: Assists patients and families with terminal illnesses; provides physical and/or psychological relief and terminal counseling.

Information and Referral Services: Furnishes care-givers with names of available service agencies or providers to meet a specific need.

Legal Services: Necessary to handle legal matters like wills, trusts, competency issues, spousal liability for payment.

Mental Health Services:	Inpatient or outpatient psychiatric, psychological, social work, and other services to help persons cope with acute and chronic emotional problems.
Occupational Therapy:	Assists with person-environment adaptation when physical or cognitive disability prevents normal adaptation, e.g., special mobility arrangements, feeding assists, restoration of physical and psychosocial function through therapeutic activity.
Paid Companion/Sitter:	Individual to stay with patient and provide supervision, some light care, and social stimulation.
Patient Assessments:	Evaluation and monitoring of person's physical, psychosocial, and functional status.
Personal Care:	Assistance with activities of daily living (bathing, eating, toileting, ambulation, etc.).
Personal Emergency Response:	Signals to a receiver outside the home (e.g., hospital, police, fire station) that the person has fallen or is in need of emergency aid.
Physical Therapy:	Assists person with rehabilitation or maintenance of physical capacities such as ambulation, transferring to toilet, eating, etc., which rely on coordination of muscles and other physical capacities (lung, cardiac, etc.). Useful with dementia patients who are unable to move about to prevent skin breakdown and pressure sores.
Physician Services:	Primary physician provides medical care and may make referrals to other providers to reduce deleterious effect of physical illness or cognitive ability.
Protective Services:	To prevent and intervene when physical, verbal, or psychological abuse is an issue.
Recreational Services:	Provide opportunities for self-expression through hobbies, interests, etc., in such a way that cognitive ability is reinforced while person enjoys him/herself and socializes with others if desired.
Respite Care:	Relief for care-giver furnished in the home, hospital, or long-term care facility by trained care-givers.
Skilled Nursing:	Usually what is meant by "nursing home" level of care in which licensed nurses are on staff in suffi-

cient numbers set by law to care for seriously disabled or ill persons.

Speech Therapy: Remediation of communication difficulties following a stroke, head injury or facilitating communication in persons with progressive, degenerative diseases involving loss of motor ability and/or cognition.

Supervision: Keeping an eye on demented persons in an individual or group setting to monitor behavior and preventing physical injury or psychosocial stress.

Telephone Reassurance: Support to care-giver or person with dementia living alone by individual(s) agreeing to do so on a regular basis. Can be used to combat isolation or to check on daily to see whether person is well.

Transportation: Getting to and from sites where needed services, shopping, and other resources are available.

Based on suggestions in US Congress, Office of Technology Assessment, *Losing a Million Minds: Confronting the Tragedy of Alzheimer's Disease and Related Disorders and Other Dementias*, OTA-BA-323 (Washington, DC, US Government Printing Office, April, 1987).

It is a good idea for the counselor who wishes to refer to and/or coordinate services as part of their intervention to obtain and maintain a current listing of resources for each service available in the local community. Good sources of such information include: the Area Agency on Aging, local Alzheimer's Association chapter, local Information Line (United Way is a typical local sponsor of such a service), state and regional professional groups, and hospital-sponsored referral services.

Notes

Chapter 1

1. C. Colarusso and R. Nemiroff. *Adult Development* (New York: Plenum Press, 1981), p. 201.
2. Ibid., p. 199.
3. H. Maier. *Three Theories of Child Development* (New York: Harper & Row, 1969), p. 71.
4. Ibid., p. 72.
5. A. Verwoerdt. *Clinical Geropsychiatry, 2nd ed.* (Baltimore: Williams and Wilkins Co., 1981), p. 13.
6. Maier. *Child Development*, p. 72.
7. M. Lewis and J. Brooks. "Infants' social perception: a constructionist view." In L. Cohen and P. Salapatek, eds., *Perception of Space, Speech, and Sound*, vol. 3 of *Infant Perception: From Sensation to Cognition* (New York: Academic Press, 1975), p. 101–48.
8. M. Lewis and R. Butler. "Life review therapy: Putting memories to work in individual and group psychotherapy." *Geriatrics*, pp. 29, 165–73, 1974.
9. E. Cohen. "History of services for the memory-impaired elderly." In L. Hiatt, N. Merlino, and J. Ronch, eds., *Innovations in the Care of the Mentally Impaired Elderly:* Conference proceedings (Albany: New York State Department of Health, 1987), p. 7.
10. D. Cohen, G. Kennedy, and C. Eisdorfer. "Phases of change in the patient with Alzheimer's dementia: A conceptual dimension for defining health-care management." *Journal of the American Geriatrics Society*, 32, 1 (1984): 11–15.
11. Ibid., p. 12.
12. Ibid., p. 13.
13. Cohen. *The Mentally Impaired Elderly*, p. 13.
14. D. Cohen, et al., p. 14.
15. Ibid.

Chapter 2

1. Hiatt et al, *Innovations in the Care of The Mentally Impaired Elderly*.
2. N. Mace and P. Rabins. *The Thirty-six Hour Day* (Baltimore: The Johns Hopkins University Press, 1981).

3. D. Cohen and C. Eisdorfer. *The Loss of Self. A Family Resource for the Care of Alzheimer's Disease and Related Disorders* (New York, Plume Publishing Company, 1986).
4. L. Powell and K. Courtice. *Alzheimer's Disease: A Guide for Families* (Reading, MA: Addison Wesley Publishing Company, 1983).
5. C. Leroux. "Alzheimer's Disease Steals the Aging Mind." *Chicago Tribune*, September 1981.
6. B. Glaze. Quoted in ibid.
7. S. Zarit, N. Orr, and J. Zarit. *The Hidden Victims of Alzheimer's Disease: Families under Stress* (New York: New York University Press, 1985).
8. C. Simon. "A Care Package." *Psychology Today*, 22, 4 April 1988, pp. 42–49.
9. J. Spikes. "Grief, Death, and Dying." In E. W. Busse and D. Blazer, eds., *Handbook of Geriatric Psychiatry* (New York: Van Nostrand Reinhold, 1980), p. 420.
10. M. Roach. *Another Name for Madness* (Boston: Houghton Mifflin, 1985), p. 179.
11. B. Rovner, introduction to M. Doernberg, *Stolen Mind* (Chapel Hill: Algonquin Books, 1986), p. 14.
12. M. Roach. Introduction: "Another Name for Madness." In A. Kalicki, ed., *Confronting Alzheimer's Disease* (Owings Mills, MD: National Health Publishing, 1987), p. 14.
13. Ibid.
14. Roach, *Another Name for Madness*, p. 14.
15. Mace and Rabins, *The Thirty-six Hour Day*, p. 164.
16. Doernberg, *Stolen Mind*, p. 84.
17. Ibid., p. 217.
18. Ibid., p. 182.
19. Ibid., p. 190.
20. E. Kubler-Ross. *On Death and Dying* (New York: MacMillan, 1969).
21. E. Erikson. *Childhood and Society* (New York: W. W. Norton, 1963), p. 268.
22. P. Wisocki and J. Averill. "The Challenge of Bereavement." In L. Cartensen and B. Edelstein, eds., *Handbook of Clinical Gerontology* (New York: Pergamon Press, 1987) p. 312.
23. Kubler-Ross. *On Death and Dying*.
24. Doernberg, *Stolen Mind*, p. 114.
25. Ibid., p. 94.
26. Ibid., p. 144.
27. Ibid.
28. Ibid.
29. Ibid., p. 145.
30. Wisocki and Averill. *The Challenge of Bereavement*, p. 313.
31. Doernberg. *Stolen Mind*, p. 179.
32. Maier. *Three Theories of Child Development*, pp. 81–158.
33. Colarusso and Nemiroff. *Adult Development*, p. 201.
34. A. Freud. *Normality and Pathology in Childhood: Assessments of Development*

(New York: International Universities Press, 1965), p. 62.
35. Colarusso and Nemiroff. *Adult Development*, pp. 201–207.
36. Doernberg. *Stolen Mind*, p. 112.
37. Erikson. *Childhood and Society*, p. 262.
38. Maier. *Child Development*, p. 61.
39. Erikson. *Childhood and Society*, p. 261.
40. Maier. *Child Development*, p. 61.
41. Doernberg. *Stolen Mind*, p. 147.
42. Ibid.
43. Maier. *Child Development*, p. 60.
44. Colarusso and Nemiroff. *Adult Development*, p. 201.
45. Ibid., p. 204.
46. Ibid., p. 204.
47. D. Guthrie. *Grandpa Doesn't Know It's Me* (New York: Human Sciences Press, 1986).
48. W. Van Ornum and J. Mordock. *Crisis Counseling with Children and Adolescents* (New York: Continuum Publishing Co., 1987), p. 68.
49. G. Pollack. "The Mourning Liberation Process: Ideas on the Inner Life of the Older Adult." In J. Sadavoy and M. Leszcz, eds., *Treating the Elderly with Psychotherapy: The Scope of Change in Later Life* (Madison, CT: International Universities Press, 1987), pp. 13–14.
50. B. Silverstone and H. Hyman. *You and Your Aging Parent* (Mt. Vernon, New York: Consumers Union, 1982), p. 46.
51. Zarit, Orr, and Zarit. *Hidden Victims of Alzheimer's Disease*, p. 114.
52. L. Steinman. "Reactivated Conflicts with Aging Parents." In P. Ragan, ed., *Aging Parents* (Los Angeles: University of Southern California Press, 1979), p. 129.
53. D. Cohen. "Management of Stress in Families Caring for Relatives with Alzheimer's Disease and Related disorders." In G. Landsberg ed., *Preventing Mental Health Problems in the Elderly: Directions and Strategies* (Nutley, NJ: Hoffman LaRoche, 1983), p. 83.
54. S. Zarit. "The burden of care-givers." In A. Kalicki, ed., *Confronting Alzheimer's Disease* (Owings Mills, MD: National Health Publishing, 1987), p. 115.
55. M. Roach. *Another Name for Madness*, pp. 178–79.
56. B. Rovner, introduction to M. Doernberg, *Stolen Mind*, p. 10.
57. I. Nagy and G. Spark. *Invisible Loyalties: Reciprocity in Intergenerational Family Therapy* (Hagerstown, MD: Harper & Row, 1973), p. 37.
58. E. McEwan. "The Whole Grandfather: An Intergenerational Approach to Family Therapy." In J. Sadavoy and M. Leszcz, eds., *Treating the Elderly with Psychotherapy* (Madison, CT: International Universities Press, 1987), p. 297.
59. E. Brody. "Patient care as a normative family stress." *The Gerontologist*, 25:1, 19–24, 1985.
60. E. McEwan, p. 300.

Chapter 3

1. S. Hoffman, C. Platt, K. Barry, and L. Hamill. "When Language Fails: Non-verbal Communication Abilities of the Demented." Paper presented at annual meeting, Gerontological Society of America, San Antonio, November 1984.
2. S. Hoffman, C. Platt, and K. Barry. "Comforting the Confused: The Importance of Non-verbal Communication in the Care of People with Alzheimer's Disease." *American Journal of Alzheimer's Care and Research*, January/February 1988, pp. 25–30.
3. L. Gwyther. *Care of Alzheimer's Patients: A Manual for Nursing Home Staff* (Washington, DC: American Health Care Association and the Alzheimer's Disease and Related Disorders Association, 1985).
4. Hoffman et al, "When Language Fails," p. 26.
5. Gwyther, *Care of Alzheimer's Patients*, p. 92.

Chapter 4

1. P. Alpaugh and M. Haney. *Counseling the Older Adult: A Training Manual for Para-Professionals and Beginning Counselors* (Los Angeles: The University of Southern California Press, 1978).
2. A. Comfort. *The Practice of Geriatric Psychiatry* (New York: Elsevier North Holland, Inc., 1980), p. 12.
3. J. Ronch and J. Maizler. "Individual Psychotherapy with the Institutionalized Elderly." *American Journal of Orthopsychiatry*, 47:275–83, 1977.
4. Comfort. *Geriatric Psychiatry*, pp. 68–69.
5. Alpaugh and Haney. *Counseling the Older Adult*, p. 19.
6. O. Sacks. *The Man Who Mistook His Wife for a Hat* (New York: Summit Books, 1985), p. 37.
7. L. Powell and K. Courtice. *Alzheimer's Disease: A Guide for Families* (Reading, MA: Addison-Wesley Publishing Co., 1983), p. 137.

Chapter 5

1. J. Marmor. *Psychiatry in Transition* (New York: Bruner-Mazel, 1974).
2. A. Goldfarb. "A psychosocial and sociophysiological approach to aging." In N. E. Zinberg and I. Kaufman, eds., *Normal Psychology of the Aging Process* (New York: International Universities Press, 1978), p. 69.

Chapter 6

1. Zarit, Orr, and Zarit. *The Hidden Victims of Alzheimer's Disease*, p. 73.
2. N. Mace. "The Family" in US Congress Office of Technology Assess-

ment. *Losing a Million Minds: Confronting the Tragedy of Alzheimer's Disease and Other Dementias* OTA BA-323 (Washington, DC: US Government Printing Office, April 1987), p. 137.
3. Mace and Rabins, *The Thirty-six Hour Day.*
4. L. H. Snyder, P. Rupprecht, J. Pyrek, S. Brekhus, and T. Moss. "Wandering." *The Gerontologist*, 18:3, 1978.
5. L. G. Hiatt. "The Happy Wanderer." *Nursing Homes*, 29:2, 27–31, 1980.
6. Ibid.
7. T. Cornbleth. "Effects of a Protected Hospital Ward Area on Wandering and Nonwandering Geriatric Patients." *Journal of Gerontology*, 32, (1977) 5:573–77.
8. Hiatt. "Happy Wanderer," p. 28.
9. Snyder et al, "Wandering," p. 276.
10. Mace and Rabins. *The Thirty-six Hour Day*, p. 91.
11. L. Hiatt. "Happy Wanderer," p. 28.
12. Mace and Rabins. *The Thirty-six Hour Day*, p. 91.
13. Hiatt. "Happy Wanderer," p. 28.
14. E. Goffman. *Asylums: Essays on the Social Situation of Mental Patients and Other Inmates* (New York: Anchor Books, 1961), p. 6.
15. Snyder et al, "Wandering," p. 276.
16. J. Rader. "A comprehensive staff approach to problem wandering." *The Gerontologist*, 27:6 1987, p. 758.
17. Snyder et al., "Wandering," p. 280.
18. Rader. *The Gerontologist*, p. 758.
19. N. Hindlian. "Case Histories of Wandering." *American Journal of Alzheimer's Care and Research*, January–February 1988, p. 38.
20. Verwoerdt. *Clinical Geropsychiatry*, p. 100.
21. J. Cohen-Mansfield and N. Billig. "Agitated Behaviors in the Elderly: 1. A conceptual review." *Journal of the American Geriatrics Society*, 34 (October 1986): 10, 711–21.
22. J. Cohen-Mansfield. "Agitated Behaviors in the Elderly: 2. Preliminary Results in the Cognitively Deteriorated." *Journal of the American Geriatrics Society*, 34(1986) 10, 722–27.
23. Ibid.
24. Ibid.
25. J. Ronch, panel presentation, "Assessment." In L. Hiatt, N. Merlino, and J. Ronch, eds., *Innovations in the Care of the Memory Impaired Elderly*: Conference Proceedings (Albany, NY: State Department of Health, 1987, p. 54.
26. L. G. Hiatt. "Disorientation Is More Than a State of Mind." *Nursing Homes*, 29, 4(1980): 30–36.
27. K. Goldstein. "Functional Disturbances in Brain Damage." In S. Arieti, ed., *American Handbook of Psychiatry*, 1:39, pp. 770–93 (New York: Basic Books, 1959).
28. N. Mace. "The Family," p. 137.

29. Gwyther. *Care of Alzheimer's Patients,* p. 68.
30. Ibid.
31. J. Piaget and B. Inhelder. *The Psychology of the Child* (New York: Basic Books, 1969), p. 13.
32. Gwyther. *Care of Alzheimer's Patients,* pp. 70–71.
33. Doernberg. *Stolen Mind,* p. 108.
34. Mace and Rabins. *The Thirty-six Hour Day,* p. 101.
35. N. Mace. "The Family," p. 137.
36. N. Mace and P. Rabins, p. 102.
37. Ibid., p. 100.
38. R. L. Kahn. "The Mental Health System and the Future Aged." *The Gerontologist,* 15:1, 24–31, 1975.
39. A. Verwoerdt. *Clinical Geropsychiatry,* p. 46.
40. Ibid., p. 84.
41. Ibid., p. 95.
42. E. Rubin, W. Drevets, and W. Burke. "The Nature of Psychotic Symptoms in Senile Dementia of the Alzheimer's Type." *Journal of Geriatric Psychiatry and Neurology,* 1:1, 1988, pp. 16–20.
43. Mace and Rabins. *The Thirty-six Hour Day,* p. 99.
44. P. Ostergaard. "Capgras Syndrome in Senile Dementia of the Alzheimer Type." *Journal of the American Geriatrics Society,* 33:11, 1985, p. 811.

Chapter 7

1. US Congress, Office of Technology Assessment. *Losing a Million Minds,* p. 5.
2. Yankelovich, Skelly, and White, Inc. "Caregivers of Patients with Dementia," contract report prepared for the Office of Technology Assessment US Congress, 1986, cited in US Congress Office of Technology Assessment, *Losing a Million Minds,* p. 23.
3. N. Silverstein and J. Hyde. "Utilizing an existing service system to aid Alzheimer's clients and their families: The Massachusetts Home Care Network." *American Journal of Alzheimer's Care and Research,* 2:2, 1987.
4. S. Ferris, T. Crook, C. Flicker, B. Reisberg, and R. Bartus. "Assessing cognitive impairment and evaluating treatment effects: Psychometric performance tests." In L. W. Poon, ed., *Handbook for Clinical Memory Assessment of Older Adults* (Washington, DC: American Psychological Association, 1986), p. 139.
5. E. Skurla, J. Rogers, and T. Sunderland. "Direct Assessment of Activities of Daily Living in Alzheimer's Disease." *Journal of the American Geriatrics Society,* 36 (1988): 97–103.
6. J. Ronch. "Assessment." In L. Hiatt, N. Merlino, and J. Ronch, eds., *Innovations in the Care of the Mentally Impaired Elderly:* Conference Proceedings (Albany, NY: State Department of Health, 1987), p. 53.

7. J. Ronch. "Specialized Alzheimer's Units in Nursing Homes: Pros and Cons." *American Journal of Alzheimer's Care and Research*, 2:4, 1987.
8. Zarit, Orr, and Zarit. *Hidden Victims of Alzheimer's Disease*, p. 73.
9. B. L. Neugarten. "Personality and aging." In J. Birren and K. W. Schaie, eds., *Handbook of the Psychology of Aging* (Cincinnati: Van Nostrand Reinold, 1977), p. 626.
10. J. Burks and M. Rubenstein. *Temperament Styles in Adult Interaction: Applications in Psychotherapy* (New York: Bruner Mazel, 1979).
11. S. Hoffman, C. Platt, K. Barry, and L. Hamill. "When Language Fails: Non-verbal Communication Abilities of the Demented." Paper presented at annual meeting, Gerontological Society of America, San Antonio, November 1984.
12. J. Ronch. "Prevention: The Role of Long-Term Care Facilities." In G. Landsberg, ed., *Preventing Mental Health Problems in the Elderly: Directions and Strategies* (Nutley, NJ: Hoffman-LaRoche, 1983), p. 53.

Chapter 8

1. Zarit, Orr, and Zarit. *The Hidden Victims of Alzheimer's Disease*, p. 73.
2. S. Ferris, G. Steinberg, E. Shulman, and R. Kahn. "Institutionalization of Alzheimer's-Disease Patients: Precipitating Factors and Effects of Intervention and Counseling." Final report AARP Ardrus Foundation (Department of Psychiatry, New York University Medical Center, 1987).
3. E. Colerick and L. George. "Predictors of Institutionalization Among Care-givers of Patients with Alzheimer's Disease." *Journal of the American Geriatrics Society*, 43(1986): 493–98.
4. N. Mace. "Programs and Services That Specialize in the Care of Persons with Dementia." In US Congress Office of Technology Assessment, *Losing a Million Minds*, p. 241.
5. Hiatt, Merlino, and Ronch, eds., *Innovations in the Care of the Mentally Impaired Elderly*.
6. Mace. *Losing a Million Minds*, p. 241.
7. US Congress Office of Technology Assessment, *Losing a Million Minds*, p. 254.
8. Ibid.
9. Ibid.
10. Hiatt, Merlino, and Ronch. *Care of the Mentally Impaired Elderly*, p. 2.
11. US Congress, *Losing a Million Minds*, p. 3.
12. Ibid., p. 244.
13. J. Ronch. "Specialized Alzheimer's Units in Nursing Homes: Pros and Cons." *American Journal of Alzheimer's Care and Research*, 2:4, 1987.
14. A. Weiner and J. Reingold. Letter to *Hospital and Community Psychiatry*, 37:8, 1987, p. 845.
15. D. Benson, D. Cameron, E. Humback, L. Servino, and S. Gambert. "Es-

tablishment and Impact of a Dementia Unit Within a Nursing Home." *Journal of the American Geriatrics Society,* 35(1987): 319–23.
16. A. Weiner. "A Nationwide Survey of Special Units." In A. Kalicki, ed., *Confronting Alzheimer's Disease* (Owings Mills, MD: National Health Publishing, 1987), pp. 80–108.
17. Ronch. "Specialized Alzheimer's Units," p. 13.
18. Mace. *Losing a Million Minds,* p. 259.
19. W. Wolfensberger. "An overview of social role valorization and some reflections on elderly mentally retarded persons." In M. Janicki and H. Wisniewski, eds., *Aging and Developmental Disabilities* (Baltimore: Paul H. Brookes Publishing Co., 1985), p. 61.
20. Ibid.
21. B. Esposito. "Support services for families." In A. Kalicki, ed., *Confronting Alzheimer's Disease,* pp. 120–32.
22. B. Rovner, introduction to M. Doernberg, *Stolen Mind,* p. 14.
23. R. Vickers. "The elderly." In A. Kraft, ed., *Psychiatry: A Concise Textbook for Primary Care Practice* (New York, Arco Medical Publishers, 1977), pp. 187–208.
24. D. Axelrod. "The Roots of Innovation." In Hiatt, Merlino, and Ronch, *Care of the Mentally Impaired Elderly,* p. 17.
25. R. L. Kahn. "The Mental Health System and the Future Aged." *The Gerontologist,* 15:1, 23–31, 1975.
26. Silverstone and Hyman. *You and Your Aging Parent,* p. 47.
27. S. Tobin and M. Lieberman. *Last Home for the Aged* (San Francisco: Jossey-Bass, 1976), p. 7.
28. J. Marks. New York City Chapter A.D.R.D.A. personal communication, 1987.
29. Silverstone and Hyman. *You and Your Aging Parent,* p. 204.
30. J. Blass. "Pragmatic pointers on managing the demented patient." *Journal of the American Geriatrics Society,* 34(1986): 548–49.
31. J. Ronch. "Specialized Alzheimer's Units," p. 13.

Appendix A

1. R. Katzman. "Alzheimer's Disease: Advances and Opportunities." *Journal of the American Geriatrics Society,* 35(1987): 69–73.
2. US Congress Office of Technology Assessment, *Losing a Million Minds: Confronting the Tragedy of Alzheimer's Disease and Other Dementias* OTA-BA 323 (Washington, DC: US Government Printing Office, April 1987).
3. Ibid.
4. L. H. Snyder, P. Rupprecht, J. Pyrek, S. Brekhus and T. Moss. "Wandering." *The Gerontologist,* 1:3, 1978.
5. M. Raskind and M. Storrie. "The Organic Mental Disorders." In E. W. Busse and D. Blazer, eds., *Handbook of Geriatric Psychiatry* (New York, Van-Nostrand Reingold Co., 1980), p. 305.

6. Ibid.
7. M. Roth. "Diagnosis of Senile Dementia." In R. Katzman, R. Terry, and K. Bick, eds., *Alzheimer's Disease: Senile Dementia and Related Disorders* (New York, Raven Press, 1978).
8. Raskind and Storrie. "Organic Mental Disorders."
9. Ibid.
10. R. C. Young, M. W. Manley, and G. S. Alexopolous. "I Don't Know: Responses in Elderly Depressives and in Dementia." *Journal of the American Geriatrics Society*, 33(1985): 253.
11. D. Blazer. *Depression in Late Life* (St. Louis: C. V. Mosby Company, 1982).
12. Adapted from B. Gurland and J. Toner. "Differentiating Dementia from Nondementing Conditions." In R. Mayeux and W. Rosen, eds., *Advances in Neurology*, vol. 38, "The Dementias" (New York: Raven Press, 1983), pp. 1–17.
13. N. L. Mace and P. Rabins. *The Thirty-six Hour Day* (Baltimore, MD: The Johns Hopkins University Press, 1981).
14. National Institutes of Health Consensus Development Conference Statement 6:11, July 6–8, 1987.
15. US Congress, *Losing A Million Minds*.
16. G. Blessed, B. E. Tomlinson, and M. Roth. "The Association Between Quantitative Measures of Dementia and of Senile Change in the Cerebral Grey Matter of Elderly Subjects." *British Journal of Psychiatry*, 114(1968): 797–811.
17. B. Reisberg, S. H. Ferris, and T. Crook. "Signs, Symptoms, and Course of Age-Associated Cognitive Decline." In K. L. Davis, J. H. Growdon, E. Usdin, and R. J. Wurtman, eds., *Alzheimer's disease: A Report of Progress in Research* (New York: Raven, 1982).
18. L. Gwyther. *Care of Alzheimer's Patients: A Manual for Nursing Home Staff*, Washington, DC, The American Health Care Association and the Alzheimer's Disease and Related Disorders Association, 1985.
19. The Burke Rehabilitation Center *Managing the Person with Intellectual Loss at Home*, White Plains, NY, 1980.
20. B. V. Reifler, G. B. Cox, R. J. Hanley. "Problems of Mentally Ill Elderly As Perceived By Patients, Families, and Clinicians." *The Gerontologist*, 21, 165, 1981.

Bibliography

Alzheimer's Disease and Related Disorders

A. General

US Congress Office of Technology Assessment. *Losing a Million Minds: Confronting the Tragedy of Alzheimer's Disease and Related Disorders and Other Dementias* OTA-BA-323. Washington, DC; US Government Printing Office, April 1987.

B. Clinical Aspects (Technical volumes for professionals)

Bayles, K., and Kaszniak, A. *Communication and Cognition in Normal Aging and Dementia.* Boston: Little Brown Company, 1987.
Corkin, S., Davis, K., Growdon, J., Usdin, E., and Wurtman, R., eds., *Alzheimer's Disease: A Report of Progress in Research.* New York: Raven Press, 1982.
Gilhooly, M., Zarit, S., and Birren, J., eds., *The Dementias: Policy and Management.* Englewood Cliffs, NJ: Prentice-Hall, 1986.
Mayeux, R., and Rosen, W., eds. *Advances in Neurology.* Vol. 38, *The Dementias.* New York: Raven Press, 1983.
Miller, N., and Cohen, G., eds., *Clinical Aspects of Alzheimer's Disease and Senile Dementias.* New York: Raven Press, 1981.
Reisberg, B., *Alzheimer's Disease: The Standard Reference.* New York: The Free Press, 1983.

C. Family Oriented and Care-related

Carroll, David L. *When Your Loved One Has Alzheimer's A Caregiver's Guide Based on Methods Developed by The Brookdale Center on Aging.* New York: Harper & Row, 1989.
Cohen, D., and C. Eisdorfer. *The Loss of Self: A Family Resource for the Care of Alzheimer's Disease and Related Disorders.* New York: N.A.L. Plume Books, 1986.
Mace, N., and P. Rabins. *The Thirty-six Hour Day.* Baltimore, MD: The Johns Hopkins University Press, 1981.

Oliver, R., and F. Bock. *Coping with Alzheimer's: A Caregivers Emotional Survival Guide.* New York: Dodd, Mead and Company, 1987.

Powell, L., and K. Courtice. *Alzheimer's Disease: A Guide for Families.* Reading, MA: Addison-Wesley, 1983.

D. Institutional-oriented and Care-related.

Gwyther, L. *Care of Alzheimer's Patients: A Manual for Nursing Home Staff.* Washington, DC: The American Health Care Association and the Alzheimer's Disease and Related Disorders Association, 1985.

Journals

1. *The American Journal of Alzheimer's Care and Research*
2. *Clinical Gerontologist*
3. *The Gerontologist*
4. *Journal of the American Geriatrics Society*
5. *The Journal of Geriatric Psychiatry and Neurology*
6. *Journal of Gerontological Nursing*
7. *Journal of Social Work and Aging*

Newsletters and Information

Alzheimer's Association
70 E. Lake St.
Chicago, Illinois 60601
(1-800-621-0379) (In Illinois 1-800-621-0379)
Local chapters also may publish a newsletter. Consult with National A.D.R.D.A. for address of the one nearest you.
Area Agency on Aging.

Alzheimer's Support Groups

For information about the group nearest you, contact: National Alzheimer's Association call 1-800-621-0379 (in Illinois 1-800-572-6037) for location of the chapter near you.

State Office of Aging or local area agency on aging can also direct you to local support groups.